ASSESSMENT & MANAGEMENT
OF EMOTIONAL REACTIONS TO
BRAIN DAMAGE & APHASIA

Far Communication Disorders Series

Series Editors: Chris Code and David Rowley, Department of Speech Pathology, Leicester Polytechnic, Leicester, England.

The *Far Communication Disorders Series* aims to provide books in speech and language pathology and therapy for the clinician and student clinician. Each book in the series will aim to be practical, readable and affordable. Currently available and forthcoming titles include:

Parents, Families, and the Stuttering Child
Edited by Lena Rustin

Treating Phonological Disorders in Children. Metaphon - Theory to Practice
Janet Howell & Elizabeth Dean

Assessment and Management of Emotional and Psychosocial Reactions to Aphasia and Brain Damage
Peter Währborg

Group Encounters in Communication Disorders
Edited by Margaret Fawcus

Management of Acquired Aphasia in Children
Janet Lees

The Clinician's Guide to Linguistic Profiling of Language Impairment
Martin J Ball

Cluttering: A Clinical Perspective
Edited by Florence Myers & Kenneth O St Louis

Computers in Management and Therapy
Edited by David Rowley & Chris Code

Introductory Guide to Clinical Syntactic Analysis
Eeva Lainonen & Susan Fasler

Which Screen? A User's Guide to Speech and Language Screening Tests
Joanne Corcoran

Far Communication Disorders Series

ASSESSMENT & MANAGEMENT OF EMOTIONAL REACTIONS TO BRAIN DAMAGE & APHASIA

Peter Währborg PhD, MD

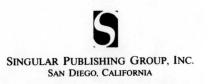

SINGULAR PUBLISHING GROUP, INC.
SAN DIEGO, CALIFORNIA

Copyright 1991 by **Far Communications Ltd., 5 Harcourt Estate, Kibworth, Leics. LE8 0NE, Great Britain** (Tel. 0533 796166)

British Library Cataloguing in Publication Data:

Währborg, Peter
Assessment and management of emotional and psychosocial reactions to brain damage and aphasia.
1. Aphasia
I. Title.
616.855206

ISBN 0 9514728-3-6

Published and Distributed in the United States and Canada by
Singular Publishing Group Inc.,
4284 41st. St.,
San Diego,
California 92105

ISBN 1-879105-18-7

Printed and Bound in Great Britain by
BPCC Wheatons Ltd., Exeter.

CONTENTS

Preface   *vii*

Chapter 1   1
Introduction

Chapter 2   5
Aphasia and Behaviour

Chapter 3   32
Aphasia and the Family

Chapter 4   40
Towards a Model of Psychological Reactions to Brain Damage and Aphasia

Chapter 5   49
The Assessment of Emotional and Psychosocial Disorder
in Aphasic Individuals and Their Families

Chapter 6   70
Management and Treatment of Psychological and Social Problems
in Aphasics and Their Families

Chapter 7   98
Long-term Evolution of Psychosocial and Emotional State

References   104

Index   113

Dedication

to
Stina Linell
the Grand Old Lady of Swedish Aphasiology
who cares so much

Over the centuries physicians and psychologists have studied brain and behaviour relationships with different methods and with varying purposes. Cultural, political and social attitudes have influenced the direction of these studies and also progress in the different basic subject areas that contribute to the understanding of this complex field.

The purpose of this book is to contribute to the understanding of emotional, behavioural and social reactions after onset of brain damage and aphasia. It is written for clinicians and students in speech pathology, logopedics, psychology and medicine but will be of interest to anyone who is interested in the field. I hope that it will prove useful to all these professionals working with brain damaged individuals.

I wish to express my warm thanks to Dr Chris Code who asked me to write this book. I also want to express my sincere gratitude to Dr Peter Borenstein and his wife Dr Eva Hedberg-Borenstein who has shared with me so much of their profound knowledge in the field. For some years now we have been working together in Gothenburg and it is my hope that we will continue to do so in the future. They have also been kind enough to read an early draft and made valuable suggestions. I also acknowledge a debt to Lisbeth who has struggled with me as well as the manuscript. I can repay only with gratitude and love.

Gothenburg
September 1990

Peter Wåhrborg

Chapter 1

Introduction

Head injuries resulting in loss of speech and other functions were reported in ancient Egypt. The Egyptian surgeons claimed in the "Edwin Smith's papyrus" (3.500 b.c.) that the loss of speech was caused by *the breath of an outside god or death* and that the patient *was silent in sadness*. Loss of language ability, or aphasia, has been described by many authors since then. An early and interesting observation was made in 1745 by Olof Dahlin, a member of the Swedish Academy of Science. He described a man who suffered from paralysis of the right side of his body and a complete loss of speech after a sudden onset of illness. Even after two years he was still not able to speak, but he was able to sing a few hymns if he got some help in starting.

Acquired aphasia can be defined as an impaired ability to use language due to brain damage. The etiology is a cerebrovascular accident (CVA) in 85 per cent of the cases (Höök 1979). In the rest neoplasm, trauma, infection, degenerative disorders, or more rarely, multiple sclerosis or a cerebral abscess are found. While the incidence of CVA or stroke has been reported as declining in the USA (Soltero, Kiang Liu, Cooper, Stamlel and Garside 1978), there have been reports indicating an increasing incidence of brain injuries (Kurtzke 1982). In a report by Apt and Kitzing (1987) the incidence of CVA in Sweden has been calculated as 200 per 10,000 inhabitants per year. The incidence of aphasia was reported to be 50 per 10,000 inhabitants (Mean = 49.3) per year. Of these cases about 50 per cent were referred to speech therapy.

Systematic study of aphasia began to evolve in the 19th. century (for recent introductions see Caplan 1987; Code 1989; Murdoch 1990). In 1861 Paul Broca described a patient who had lost the faculty of speech. After performing a post-mortem study he concluded that the patient's problems were due to the lesion he found in the posterior portion of the inferior frontal gyrus, thereafter called Broca's

Area. Another step forward was taken in 1874 when Carl Wernicke published data confirming the existence of another form of aphasia with fluent speech and impaired comprehension. Wernicke claimed that the comprehension disorder was associated with a lesion in the posterior portion of the superior temporal gyrus, now called Wernicke's Area. He distinguished between two separate types of aphasia, motor and sensory. He also postulated a third variety of aphasia, conduction aphasia, based upon a diagrammatic outline of portions of the brain participating in language function. The chief symptom in conduction aphasia was paraphasia affecting phoneme production, and it was due to an interruption of fibre tracts connecting the auditory area and the motor speech area. The theories of Wernicke were developed by Lichtheim (1885) who postulated five interconnected cortical centres, four of these concerned with language (see Figure 1).

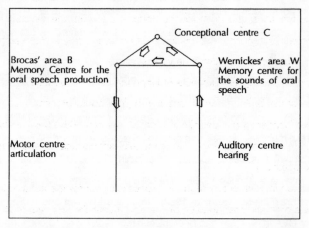

Figure 1: The Wernicke - Lichtheim model for the neurology of language.

The aphasias derived from the Wernicke-Lichtheim model: **Broca's aphasia**: lesion to **B**, disturbance in expression (nonfluent) with preserved comprehension; **Wernicke's aphasia**: lesion to **M**, disturbance in comprehension and fluent expression; **Conduction aphasia**: (Leitungsaphasie): disconnection **W - B**, normal comprehension, fluent speech and disturbance in repetition; **Transcortical sensory aphasia**: disconnection **W - C**, disturbed comprehension, normal spontaneous speech, normal repetition; **Transcortical motor aphasia**: disconnection **C - B**, normal comprehension, nonfluent speech, normal in repetition.

Introduction

The contributions of Wernicke and Lichtheim constitute the beginnings of the comprehensive development of aphasiology. During the following decades important contributions were made by many others including Liepmann, Freud, Kleist, Goldstein, Dejerine, Bastian, Jackson, Marie, Head and Luria. Different taxonomies were developed, based on different observations and there are several important contemporary models. In this book we will use the Bostonian taxonomy which is based on the classical Wernicke-Lichtheim model as a basis for discussion, mainly because of its universal usage. The main clinical features or symptoms for the classification of aphasia according to this taxonomy is verbal fluency in spontaneous speech, comprehension, oral repetition ability, confrontation naming and the presence or absence of paraphasia (Goodglass and Kaplan 1972; for detailed discussion see Caplan 1987). The model allows a clinical-neuropathologic analysis of disturbances in language functions and provides the aphasia therapist, the psychologist or the physician, useful insight into the relationships between brain and language and the general organization of the central nervous system.

Processing of the linguistic aspects of language seem to be lateralized to the left hemisphere of the brain in 99% of cases in right-handers (Benson and Geschwind 1983). In left-handers it has been found that 50 per cent with aphasia have a lesion in the left hemisphere suggesting that some left-handers use both hemispheres for language processing.

Aphasia is an impairment of linguistic processing, but for the aphasic individual it also means a dramatic change to emotional and mental life. Emotional, motivational, behavioural and social changes occur, sometimes as a result of conscious choices and sometimes through unconscious processes. Often accompanying the communication handicap is a physical handicap which limits the aphasic individual's life irrespective of wishes and choices. Not only does the aphasic person suffer a cerebral infarction, but also an "ego" infarction - the lesion also has an impact on the "self" of the patient. Aphasia is an insult in one's personal life. This book aims to discuss emotional and related problems in aphasic individual's as well as in their families. While our discussion will attempt to be scientific and the adequacy of methodological will feature to some extent, we should however, recognise that emotional and psychosocial dynamics are not only difficult to measure objectively, there very definition in problematic. Hence the difficulties inherent in clinical research on the mental, emotional and interactional consequences of aphasia.

Chapter 2

Aphasia and Behaviour

The feelings associated with a sudden onset of a hemiparesis and/or speechlessness are difficult for us to grasp. Hamilton Cameron (1959) has experienced these feelings. He will introduce this chapter in his own words:

> *It was about seven o'clock ..... when I awakened. I had no sensation of pain. I simply awakened and came to realization that during the night I suffered a paralytic aphasic stroke. I could not talk. I was immovable and I had a fantastic sensation of being enveloped in a leather bag moulded to my body. Then came a radical sensation of torturous fear, an almost indefinable sense of terror. I was in agony in my despair. I was a prey to the incubus of impending death.*

In this chapter the behavioural changes seen in aphasic persons will be described and discussed. In order to understand the individual differences in reactions and the meaning of what we observe, some important issues have to be addressed.

The Cause of Change

Analysis of a situation that is changing with time requires description and establishment of a baseline from which to measure that change. The proverb, *the more something changes the more it remains the same*, is more than a witticism. In an artful paradox it explores the relationship between persistence and change, two words we usually consider as having diametrically opposite. Traditionally a causal model has been the major factor in shaping medical and behavioural thinking. This model has been partially successful in explaining *hard* biological data, but in the behavioural sciences the model has been questioned and criticised for being to superficial and reductionistic. Causal thinking, or determinism, tends to search for basic elements or single factors and causal relations among them.

An example of linear causal theory is single factor theory, which postulates that a disease or a disorder is a result of a single noxious factor. From a philosophical point of view, a single factor model may be based on an assumption that the causal factor is a sufficient condition; that is, the presence of the factor invariably leads to the disease or the disorder no matter what constellation of other factors may be present. A variation on the theme is the assumption that a factor can be a necessary condition. This means that the factor has to be demonstrated in a case of the disease or disorder. On the other hand the actual exposure to the noxious factor does not necessarily lead to the disease or the disorder. This methodological tradition has developed to include more sophisticated multicausal models based on empirical observations. The factors are assumed to sometimes constitute a more complex interaction with each other.

The traditional approach to science described in short above appears under different labels such as, materialism, empiricism, logical positivism, reductionism and behaviourism.

There is another *softer* approach to research, especially in psychosocial consequences to brain damage. Basic to this approach is the subjective description of immediate experiences. *Soft theorists*, or phenomenologists, are a diverse group who search for causes and explanations to phenomena; but for them the search must cover not only the environment, but the history, the genetic heritage and the subjective experience of humanity, as well as numerous other unobservables. This scientific tradition has often been labelled *hermeneutic.*

6

Scientific Methods and Psychosocial Consequences of Aphasia

Research in aphasia presents a number of methodological problems. The difficulties are of significant importance since they tend to make any *tight* scientific design difficult to carry out for a range of reasons. The very nature of aphasia - communication impairment interferes with most empirical methods normally used in behavioural research.

The impaired speech of aphasic individuals restricts their answers to questions and impaired comprehension calls for caution in the interpretation of data obtained in tests, questionnaires, etc. These obvious obstacles to research result in increased demands on the researcher: attention must be paid to the way instructions or questions are presented and the way different tasks and tests are explained to the subject. The researcher's perception of the aphasic subject's situation and capacity may affect the manner in which data is gathered, classified and analyzed.

Since few psychological tests, attitude scales or other empirical tools are developed specifically for aphasic subjects or standardized on aphasic subjects, a conventional experimental approach would not be sufficient to gain knowledge about psychological or emotional problems. On the other hand, there is the danger that the looser hermeneutic approach increases the risk of bias and subjectivity on the part of the researcher. An investigator can be tempted to be selective in collecting data guided by some prior notions or beliefs rather than objectively describing the phenomena under study. As often, the most fruitful approach to improving our knowledge of psychosocial consequences of brain damage and aphasia would seem to be a combination allowing both empirical research methods and hermeneutic interpretations. This strategy is not a short cut, but requires even more scientific sensitivity and awareness to be successful.

Some factors influencing the emotional and behavioural response to brain damage have been discussed in the literature but many have received little attention. Probably the main reason for this is the difficulties inherent in trying to tease out the factors which affect the final outcome. Our lack of knowledge reflects practical and methodological obstacles associated with research on the subject. Furthermore, the human central nervous system appears to have a sophisticated way of *hiding* changes. Von Monakow noted in 1914:

> *Any injury suffered by the brain substance will lead to a struggle for the*
> *preservation of the disrupted nervous function, and the central nervous*
> *system is always (though not always to the same degree) prepared for*
> *such a struggle.* (from Powell 1981: p 20.)

Before discussing further the factors important to the emotional response to brain injury we will explore the behavioural changes found in aphasic persons.

Behavioural Changes in Aphasic Persons

An Overview

It is not a recent finding that aphasia is often combined with behavioural changes in the patient. Organic as well as psychologically determined changes have been described in early works from this century. The issue was brought to attention by authors like Meyer (1904) and Kraepelin (1921) who recognized specific emotional disorders connected with unilateral brain damage.

In 1922 Babinski described the emotional reaction later defined as the *indifference reaction*, usually following right cerebral damage and characterized by an indifference to or minimization of symptoms, euphoria and emotional placidity. The emotional change following a left hemisphere lesion was termed *catastrophic reaction* by Goldstein (1939), who defined it as the inability of a person to cope when faced with serious defects in physical and cognitive function. The person may over-react in an anxious, aggressive manner, or even become quiet, depressed and withdrawn. Another important step towards better understanding of behavioural effects of brain injuries was taken by Bleuler (1951) who reported persistent and refractory depression following stroke.

The first systematic study designed to differentiate reactions due to right and left hemispheric lesions respectively appeared in 1972 (Gainotti 1972). Gainotti divided emotional reactions into four categories; catastrophic reaction, depressive mood, indifference reactions and other reactions. The catastrophic reaction symptoms were reported more frequently in patients with a lesion in the left hemisphere and even more significantly so if the patient was aphasic. The indifference reaction symptoms were found to correlate with a right-sided lesion, and with neglect of the contralateral (opposite side to the lesion) half of the body and space.

Most studies of emotional reactions to brain damage and aphasia with patients and of their relatives, are based upon fairly soft data; that is, clinical observations, interviews and reports by relatives. In many of the studies referred to in this chapter it has been difficult to find any theoretical rationale or explicit strategy for selection of variables to be examined.

In addition to the explorative research designed to describe clinically manifested emotional and behavioural problems connected with brain damage and aphasia, the literature also contains studies whose primary purpose has been to identify psychological obstacles to re-adaption and rehabilitation. Among these are Epsmark (1973) and Kinsella and Duffy (1978, 1979). The purpose of these studies was to clarify the incidence of adjustment difficulties after stroke in aphasic and non-aphasic patients. In the reports of Bay (1961,1962) and Mapelli (1980), not only emotional but also psychotic reactions induced by aphasia were studied. Folstein, Maiberger and McHugh (1977) compared 20 consecutively admitted stroke patients with 10 orthopaedic patients. Fifty percent of the stroke group with left hemisphere lesions were depressed and only 10% of the orthopaedic patients, were found to be depressed even though the level of functional disability was considered to be the same by the authors. Reliable and valid instruments were used (the Hamilton Rating Scale of Depression, the Visual Analogue Mood Scale, the Present State Examination and the Mini-Mental State Examination, all discussed in more detail in Chapter 5).

Ross and Rush (1981) published a much noted article on the diagnosis and neuroanatomic correlates of depression in brain damaged patients and Robinson and co-workers (for an overview see Starkstein and Robinson 1988) have published several much quoted studies on mood changes in stroke patients. These studies have added new and essential information to the study of emotional reactions after brain damage. Robinson's group have restricted their studies to depression and its nature and severity, using standardized scales of measurement and established clinical symptom criteria used by the Diagnostic and Statistical Manual of Mental Disorders (DSM-III). They also correlated these observations with CT-scan analysis. The results of these studies have attracted considerable attention. Among the findings reported, the following were especially important:

1. The frequency (30-60 per cent) and the severity of mood disorders are significantly increased during the period from six months to two years post-onset.

2. In the majority of cases, depression lasts 8 to 9 months untreated.

3. The severity of the depression was significantly correlated to the proximity of the left hemisphere lesion to the frontal pole as measured on CT-scan.

Division of Reactions to Brain Damage and Aphasia

In this chapter we divide emotional reactions to brain damage and aphasia into four sub-groups: psychiatric reactions, neurobehavioral reactions, psychosocial reactions and intellectual and cognitive reactions.

1. Psychiatric reactions are defined, according to DSM-III, as minor and major psychiatric disorders, depression and emotional reactions.

2. Neurobehavioural reactions are emotional changes believed to be induced by the brain damage *per se* and related to localization of the lesion.

3. Psychosocial reactions are defined as changes in interaction and social behaviour.

4. Intellectual and cognitive changes are those involving attitudes, beliefs and knowledge.

In the remainder of this chapter, we examine each of these categories separately. We should remember that the study of emotional and behavioural reactions accompanying aphasia - with a few important exceptions - has been characterized by the use of non-systematic observation producing highly varying findings. Thus examination of the literature provides an incomplete picture of the psychological situation of aphasic individuals.

As early as 1935 (and subsequently in 1939, 1942 and 1948) Goldstein reported a constellation of reactions to brain damage which he named *catastrophic reaction*. The syndrome includes anxiety reactions, tears, aggressive behaviour, swearing, displacement, refusal, renouncement and compensatory boasting. The catastrophic reaction was considered by Goldstein as a coping strategy for survival. Survival, stated Goldstein (1939) *becomes paramount in a pathologically changed organism!* However, the survival was characterised by disorder and inconsistency and embedded in a physical and mental shock, - a state Goldstein termed catastrophic. To begin with the phenomenon was understood as a generalized response to brain damage, but in an often cited study Gainotti (1972) claimed it to be a specific response to left brain damage and most often associated with aphasia.

Depression is the most frequently reported reaction accompanying aphasia after stroke and it was a major finding by Biorn-Hansen (1957) who also found irritability, anger, frustration, general anxiety, hostility, withdrawal and rejection to be prominent aspects of the aphasics' behaviour post stroke. Some years later, Bay (1962) described an agitation-syndrome the major symptoms of which are unrestrained excitement, gesticulation, pacing back and forth and whistling and laughing for no reason.

Friedman (1961) studied the emotional reactions of aphasic patients to their language impairment and to their interpersonal relationship problems in the context of group psychotherapy. Withdrawal, denial, projection, exaggeration, regression and fear were common findings among the aphasic participants in this study. Ullman (1962) systematically observed three hundred patients over a period of three years. The major finding in this study was depression in the aphasic patients. Taylor (1969) too reported irritability, anger and frustration and emotional lability post stroke. Subjective data reported by wives of aphasic subjects in group sessions was collected by Bardach (1969) who found depression, irritability, anger, frustration and indifference being the dominating symptoms in the aphasic individuals. Hurwitz and Adams (1972) also reported depression, and catastrophic reaction, lowered self esteem and denial, as common states in aphasics.

In the Gainotti study from 1972 one hundred and sixty patients were examined, 80 with left-sided lesions and 80 with right-sided lesions. No significant differences were found between the two groups with regard to age, educational level or etiology. There were in-group differences in etiology, with 53 with left hemispheric lesions had a vascular etiology, and 27 had a neoplastic or other lesion. Of the right hemisphere damaged group 58 had a vascular etiology and 22 had a neoplastic or other etiology. During the neuropsychological examination the patient's verbal expressions were transcribed verbatim, and any behaviour that was considered indicative of emotional reaction and mood was carefully recorded. Depression and catastrophic reaction were the main findings in the patients with a left hemispheric lesion.

Espmark (1973) presented a consecutive series of data collected through interviews and questionnaires. All of the investigated subjects were under 50 years of age, with sudden onset of vascular focal lesions and were examined on average 2.8 years post onset. Eighteen patients stated that they did not suffer from aphasia , but did not undergo a detailed assessment for aphasia. Of the 72 subjects 22 were depressed, 42 suffered from general anxiety, 38 were fatigued, 35 were emotionally labile and 30 suffered from irascibility.

Benson (1973,1980) has reported depression in aphasic patients, as well as catastrophic reaction, irritability, frustration and anger. He also reported paranoid reactions (1973), a prerequisite for which, he suggests, is a severe comprehension impairment and damage to the auditory association area in the left temporal lobe. D'Afflitti and Weitz (1974) reported data from unstructured patient-family groups indicating depression, lowered self esteem and grief in the aphasic members. In their large study Jenkins, Jimenez-Pabon, Shaw and Sefer (1975) reported confusion and

13

psychotic reactions among 13 % of aphasic patients and emotional lability in 19%. Folstein *et al* (1977) also emphasised depression as a major feature in individuals following brain damage and Glozman (1982) compared an aphasic with a control group of neurological patients without aphasia and found lowered self esteem in the aphasic group. Data were reported subjectively.

Mapelli and co-workers (1980) studied 63 patients affected by aphasia of circulatory origin and found that 36 suffered from depression. Two of the 63 were characterized by a state of *psychomotor catatonic excitement*, which the authors' interpreted as *Bonhoeffer's acute exogenous reaction* (a psychotic reaction due to exogenous factors) with catatonic symptoms. Three patients of the 63 showed paranoid reaction, 3 were agitated and 14 were indifferent.

A review of the literature by Ricco-Schwartz (1982) concluded that depression, irritability, frustration, anger, emotional lability and grief were the most important behavioural changes in aphasic patients, and more recent studies seem to confirm earlier findings.

In a study based on questionnaires to spouses Währborg and Borenstein (1988) found statistically significant changes toward decreased emotional stability, lack of initiative, increased tendency towards social isolation and decreasing sexual activity. A significant tendency towards depression was also noted. A surprising finding in this study was a significant co-variation between the spouses perception (subjective opinion) of the physical impairment of their aphasic partner and a reported tendency towards social isolation. However, no such connection was found between the actual (objective testing) physical impairment and reported tendency towards social isolation.

Robinson and co-workers (Robinson and Price 1982; Robinson, Starr and Price 1984) studied the variable of time on mood disorders in stroke patients and found an obvious co-variation between mood-disorder and time since onset - depression increased with time since onset. Währborg and Borenstein (1988b) also observed a progressive psychological deterioration in aphasic and non-aphasic stroke patients.

Aphasia and Behaviour

Significant differences between the groups were found in three variables: aphasics were more irritated, touchy and had a more degrading self-esteem.

Summary

Depression is obviously the most commonly reported affective reaction occurring in aphasic patients. It is also one of the most challenging problems in aphasia rehabilitation. For this reason we examine further the relationship between aphasia and depression next. But first, we will summarize thus far.

A remarkable variety of emotional and psychosocial changes have been reported in connection with aphasia. We must bear in mind that most studies have been purely exploratory and descriptive in nature and control subjects for comparison were not included in most. As we have seen above, depression associated with aphasia has been consistently reported. This finding is recurrent and seems reliable. Folstein *et al* (1977) reported that 50% of left hemisphere damaged patients suffered depression. Moreover a range of studies have noted an association with side of lesion and depression. Several authors also describe, variably, the so-called catastrophic reaction in aphasic individuals.

It seems likely that the depressions described in the literature differ with respect to time since onset, etiology, clinical symptoms, course of the condition and prognosis, as well as cause. Therefore, each type of depression probably requires its own form of therapy, something that has hardly been tackled at all but which we discuss in later chapters.

Emotional lability and altered social life are to be expected after revolutionary and dramatic events in life like the sudden onset of brain damage and it does not seem likely that all the observations made on aphasics' emotional status are due to the aphasia or even the brain damage itself. Some of the observations on mood change reported probably reflect the dramatically changed life situation or even premorbid personality traits of the individual, and these are the subject of discussion in later chapters.

Aphasia, Depression and the Hemispheres

As we have already noted, depression is the most commonly reported emotional disorder in aphasics and there is a predominance of left-sided lesions in cases of depression after brain damage (Gainotti 1971; Folstein *et al*. 1977; Robinson and Price 1982).

Different emotional responses to hemispheric lesions were reported in the 1930s. Alford (1933) claimed that cases with left brain damage tended to develop a definite and permanent confusion of consciousness and emotional instability. The conclusion drawn from most of these earlier studies is that the altered mood is a psychological reaction to either the impaired language function or the physical handicap or both (Thompson 1948; Fisher 1961; Benson 1979). More recent studies, however, present findings which contradict this assumption and suggest a different cause for depression following damage to the left hemisphere.

Robinson *et al* (1984) ask the question:

> *What is the nature of this association between lesion location and depression? Is it, for example, a result of left anterior lesions producing a particular impairment which secondarily leads to depression or is the depression a behaviour manifestation of neurophysiological or neurochemical changes provoked by the brain injury?* (p 563).

One view is that the normal right hemisphere is much more involved in emotional processing than the left (Schwartz *et al* 1975). As discussed earlier, damage to the left hemisphere tends to result in depression, while damage in the right hemisphere tends to result in an indifferent euphoric state, sometimes referred to as *anosognosia*. Davidson (1983) reports that normal subjects during extensive EEG recordings showed an increased activity in the left frontal region during negative emotions. These observations suggest that the right hemisphere may be responsible for negative emotions while the left hemisphere seems to be concerned with positive emotions. In the growing body of literature on hemispheric asymmetry concerning the cerebral representation of emotions there is still no convincing evidence for the superiority of the right hemisphere in emotional life (see Code 1986, 1987 for discussion). Support for the hypothesis that certain regions of the two hemispheres are differentially dominant for certain positive and negative emotions comes from a range of studies with normal subjects.

Lesions to the parietal lobes result in a variety of disturbances, the most relevant for our purposes being unilateral neglect - if the lesion is on the right, which often co-occurs with denial and other apparent disturbances in mood. The common feature is an alteration of the perception of the body form on the side contralateral to the lesion, and its relation to surrounding space; especially, in tactile and visual exploration of immediate extrapersonal space. As well as its unilateral form, neglect can occur for both sides of the body from a unilateral lesion producing global disorders affecting both sides of the body.

Unilateral neglect was characterized by Benson (1979) as inattention to one side of space and one's own body. Severity can vary from 1) a tendency to neglect one side, to 2) a lack of concern about all or parts of the body on one side to 3) an unawareness of all but major stimuli on one side, to 4) *anosognosia*, that is, manifest denial of any problems involving the entire side of the body opposite the lesion. Hécaen (1967) referred to this latter behaviour as a *pantomime of massive neglect*. A fascinating description of this phenomenon was made by Jung (1974) who described a painter whose self-portraits after the lesion were restricted to the right side of the face and the canvas. With recovery over a 12 month period, the left side of the painters own face began to be represented more in the self-portraits until the whole canvas was filled with the whole face. As pointed out this disturbance is associated with right-sided lesions in the overwhelming number of cases, but does rarely occur in left-sided lesions as well and are then a severe neurobehavioural complication in aphasia rehabilitation. The contralateral syndrome described above is most often associated with a right-sided lesion in the parietal lobe while the bilateral syndrome may occur when there is a large lesion of the right hemisphere (Mountcastle 1975). The phenomenon of neglect appears to interact in complex and little understood ways with denial and other emotional reactions and the clinician should be aware of the possible influence of the condition upon behaviour. However, since our main concern is with psychological and psychosocial consequences of aphasia no further attention will be given this otherwise interesting topic.

Different emotional reactions in patients submitted to intracarotid Sodium Amytal injection have been reported (Terzian and Cecotto 1959; Rossi and Rosadini 1967). This procedure effectively anaesthetizes one hemisphere for a few minutes. A depressive-catastrophic reaction following pharmacological inactivation of the left, and a euphoric-maniacal reaction following inactivation of the right hemisphere has been reported. But in a study by Milner (1967) in Montreal no differences in emotional reactions of the kind described by Rossi and Rosadini (1967) were observed following left- and right-hemisphere Amytal injection.

Recent studies with brain damaged subjects confirm a direct link between side of lesion and mood state. Gainotti (1972: p. 48) made the general observation that there was *a difference in the quality of emotional reactions depending on the side of the cerebral lesion*. Patients with left-sided lesions are reported to display feelings of despair, hopelessness and anger while patients with right-sided lesions develops an indifferent-euphoric reaction (Sackeim *et al* 1982). In Folstein *et al's* (1977) previously mentioned study, it was found that 50% of the patients with left-sided lesions after stroke were depressed. The corresponding figure for right-sided lesions was 40%. However, only 10% of the right hemisphere damaged patients with a physical impairment comparable to the one found in the left hemisphere damaged patients were depressed. These studies therefore indicate that left hemisphere lesions are more likely to produce depression than right-sided lesions, and depression in patients with left hemisphere lesions is more serious the closer to the frontal pole the injury is located. Depression after brain damage has also been more frequently reported in anterior than in posterior lesions of the left hemisphere (Robinson and Benson 1981; Robinson and Szetala 1981).

Support for this general finding that depression following brain damage is due to organic changes in the brain comes from the observation that neither the physical impairment, the language disturbance or the impaired social functioning have been shown to correlate with depression after stroke (Finkelstein *et al* 1982; Robinson *et al* 1984; Sinyor *et al* 1986; Währborg & Borenstein 1988).

In patients with spinal cord injuries (paraplegics/quadriplegics) the prevalence of depression has been reported to be 13% (MacDonald, Nielson and Cameron 1987). Even if the groups are not comparable from a demographic standpoint such differences support the hypothesis of a specific lesion-induced depression especially in stroke patients.

However, as we shall see later, it has been observed that psychotherapeutic programmes effectively influence depression following left-hemisphere lesions with aphasia (Borenstein *et al* 1987; Borenstein, Linell and Währborg 1987), but may be due to improvement in a *secondary* depressive reaction which developed following the initial lesion-induced depression.

Most studies on brain damage, aphasia and depression have been completed with patients after stroke and the depression observed in these patients is therefore often called **post-stroke depression**. In the following section we examine post-stroke depression in some detail.

Post-Stroke Depression

For clinical and therapeutic reasons it is important to distinguish between major post-stroke depression and reactive post-stroke depression, and we examine these separately in the following short sections.

Major Post-Stroke Depression

In accordance with the characteristics given in DSM-III, the diagnostic criteria for major depression are:

(1) Dysphoric mood or loss of interest of pleasure in all or most usual activities. The dysphoric mood is characterized by symptoms such as depression, sadness, hopelessness, and irritability. The mood disturbances are prominent and relatively persistent.

(2) Presence of at least 4 of the following symptoms nearly every day for a period of at least two weeks:
- poor appetite or significant weight loss, or increased appetite or significant weight gain;
- insomnia or hypersomnia;
- psychomotor retardation or agitation;
- decrease in sexual drive;
- fatigue or loss of energy;
- feelings of worthlessness, self-reproach, or excessive or inappropriate guilt;
- complaints or evidence of diminished ability to think or concentrate;
- recurrent thoughts of death, suicidal ideation, wishes to be dead, or suicide attempts.

(3) In some cases perceptual disturbance and altered thinking in the form of hallucinations and delusions also occur.

Aphasia and Behaviour

The pathogenesis of post-stroke depression has been suggested to be related to the proximity of the left hemisphere lesion to the frontal pole (see Starkstein and Robinson 1988). The correlation between the closeness of the brain lesions to the frontal pole and the severity of depression is thought to be because anterior lesions interrupt more catecholaminergic pathways than posterior lesions do, thereby causing a more profound drop in brain norepinephrine levels. Norepinephrine acts as a chemical transmitter between the neurons in the brain and allows the conduction of signals from one neuron to another. The norepinephrine system has been implicated in the maintenance of arousal but also in the reward system of the brain, in dreaming sleep and in the regulation of mood. What is important is that the drop in norepinephrine levels ultimately leads to the behavioural expression of depression (Robinson and Szetala 1981). In 1984 Robinson *et al.* suggested a lateralized frontal affective syndrome. In their study a right hemisphere lesion group showed a reverse trend: patients with right posterior lesions were more depressed than patients with right anterior lesions. In a study by Sinyor et al. (1986) designed to replicate and extend the findings of Robinson *et al.*, it was reaffirmed that the severity of the depression tends to increase with the proximity of the lesion to the left frontal pole. The reverse relationship (i.e. increased severity of depression in right posterior lesions) was not confirmed.

A range of chemical transmitters are active in the brain. The best mapped are the so-called monoamines -dopamine, norepinephrine (= noradrenin) and serotonin. The distribution of monoaminergic neuron systems, reproduced in a coronary section of the brain. are shown in Figure 2. As can be seen the different monoamine-containing neurons project to different regions of the brain. The norepinephrine-containing neurons are concentrated to a small area in the brain stem (locus coeruleus) and the offshoots (axons) of these neurons project to many areas in the brain such as hypothalamus and the forebrain. Dopamine-containing neurons are mainly concentrated in the region of the midbrain but also to the forebrain where they are thought to be involved in regulation of emotional responses. Serotonin (=5-HT) is a monoamine transmitter concentrated in the brain stem and the neurons of this area project to hypothalamus, thalamus and many other brain regions. This transmitter is of crucial importance in the process of sensory perception, but also in many other activities and emotions. Further discussion on the neuro-transmitters is found in Chapter 5.

Figure 2: Monoaminergic neuronsystems in the brain and the spinal cord.

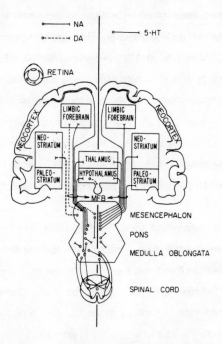

Noradrenergic (NA) and dopaminergic (DA) pathways are reproduced to the left and serotonergic pathways to the right. (Courtesy of prof. A. Carlsson, first published in 1987.)

Aphasia and Behaviour

Major post-stroke depression has been shown to be significantly associated with failure to suppress serum cortisol production following dexamethasone administration (Lipsey *et al* 1985; Reding *et al* 1985). This finding is important since it indicates a significant difference between major post-stroke depression and reactive post-stroke depression. This is also further discussed in Chapter 5.

Reactive Post-Stroke Depression

Reactive post-stroke depression refers to the psychogenetic etiology of the post-stroke syndrome; the secondary reaction to the awareness of the loss of language and other functions (cf. Thompson 1948). This natural reaction is also found in other handicap-groups and in their relatives following traumatic life events. Diagnostic criteria are in accordance with the characteristics of dysthymia given in DSM-III. The time limits given in the definition are not appropriate in this context for obvious reasons:

(1) Depressed mood for most of the day, more days than not, as indicated either by subjective account or observation by others, for at least two years.

(2) Presence, while depressed, of at least two of the following:
- poor appetite or overeating;
- insomnia or hypersomnia;
- low energy or fatigue;
- low self-esteem
- poor concentration or difficulty making decisions;
- feelings of hopelessness.

(3) During a two year period (post-stroke period) of the disturbance, never without the symptoms in (1) for more than two months at a time.

Comparison of these criteria with those for major depression in the previous section show that while the symptoms are the same, **the intensity and severity** of major depression coupled with its chronicity distinguishes it from the reactive form. Nonetheless, distinguishing between these forms - essential before meaningful therapy can begin, is far from easy. The importance of distinguishing between the two forms of post-stroke depression is emphasized by the fact that major post-stroke depression is a life-threatening disorder, since suicide is not an uncommon consequence. Differential diagnosis is further discussed in Chapter 5.

Parikh *et al* (1987) have reported a natural course lasting one year in severe post-stroke depression, while minor reactive depression has a more prolonged duration. However, in a phenomenological comparison between major post-stroke depression and what the authors termed *functional* depression, which we can read as reactive, Lipsey *et al* (1986) found that the depressive syndrome profiles in the two patient groups were highly similar. This finding can be interpreted as contradicting the frontal pole hypothesis. It is well-known that damage to the frontal lobes results in dynamic motor disturbances clinically similar to the psychomotor retardation seen in major depression. The observed similarity in the study referred to above, where all 43 patients were fulfilling the criteria for major depression, might merely be an observed similarity in behaviour between frontal lobe damaged patients and depressed patients. In other words, there are clinically important similarities in behaviour between the patients with frontal damage with and without genuine depression. Studies taking this into account would therefore be needed before the question is resolved.

The noted prolonged duration of minor or reactive depression might result from a gradual onset which reflects the individual's growing awareness of the implications of the handicap. This interpretation supports a psychological basis for the etiology of reactive depression post-stroke.

It is not surprising to find depression in survivors of stroke. What is surprising, however, is the lack of attempts at treatment reported. Fiebel *et al* (1979) reported that although one-third of 113 post-stroke patients who were followed for six months reported depression, only one patient received antidepressant medication and only one patient was referred for psychiatric treatment. At least contributing to the prevailing therapeutic neglect is uncertainty in the diagnosis and differential diagnosis of post-stroke depression and our limited understand of its nature.

The nosological considerations discussed above suggest fundamental differences between at least two subtypes of post-stroke depression requiring different therapeutic approaches. In the small body of work on treatment, both tricyclic antidepressant medication and psychotherapeutic programmes have produced optimistic results. Future studies are necessary not only to provide more detailed description of the post-stroke depression syndromes but also to identify methods which will examine the relationships between the cause of the depression and specific treatment programmes. This problem is further discussed in Chapter 6.

A range of procedures that aid examination of affective state and provide some basis for differential diagnosis are described in Chapter 5. Chapter 7 discusses approaches to intervention for individuals and families with major post-stroke and reactive depression.

Neurobehavioural Reactions in Aphasic Patients

It is sometimes difficult to distinguish between what we have classified as psychiatric reactions to brain damage and aphasia in the previous section and neurobehavioural reactions. **Neurobehavioural reactions, or *primary* reactions, are those clearly and demonstrably connected to a lesion site.** Indifference reactions, catastrophic reactions and even depressions are partly related to lesion site but do not fulfil the criteria of a *pure* neurobehavioural syndrome. They are therefore discussed under the psychiatric heading. We will now take a closer look at the intimate relationship between brain, emotions and behaviours and try to identify the neurobehavioural disorders that can to be found in aphasic patients.

Emotions and The Brain

At the turn of the century the question of emotions and their relationship to the brain was brought under consideration, especially by William James. In a classical paper *What is an emotion?* in Mind (1884) he argued in a rather provocative manner for a more brain-oriented view on emotions:

> *The physiologists who, during the past few years, have been so industriously exploring the functions of the brain, have limited their attempts at explanation to its cognitive and volitional performances. Dividing the brain into sensorial and motor centres, they have found their division to be exactly paralleled by the analysis made by empirical psychology, of the perceptive and volitional parts of the mind into their simplest elements. But the aesthetic sphere of the mind, its longings, its pleasures and pains, and its emotions, have been so ignored in all these researches that one is tempted to suppose that if either Dr Ferrier or Dr Munk were asked for a theory in brain-terms of the latter mental facts, they might both reply, either that they had as yet bestowed no thought upon the subjects, or that they had found it so difficult to make distinct hypotheses, that the matter lay for them among the problems of the future, only to be taken up after the simpler ones of the present should have been definitively solved (p. 188).*

James argued that emotions were the brain's experience of bodily changes: I cry, therefore I must be sad. His theories never became confirmed but he was without doubt a vigorous pioneer in the field. It has been known for some time that people with high cervical spinal cord transections still experienced emotions (Dana 1921). Although according to James' theories it is impossible for the brain of an individual with such damage to experience bodily change.

An opponent of James, Walter Cannon (1927), argued that the thalamus was the most important structure for emotions. Later Bard (1934) demonstrated the importance of the hypothalamus in emotional expressions and in 1937 Papez pointed to the circuit of connected forebrain structures that now bears his name (Papez Circuit, what we now refer to most commonly as the limbic system) as primarily responsible for regulations of emotions.

Modern knowledge provides us with a somewhat more complex model of human emotional life. Emotions are regarded as a function of deliberation between cortical and limbic system activities. Cortical systems produce an appropriate cognitive set that becomes emotionally coloured and motivationally meaningful when entering the limbic system.

The hypothalamus is strongly influenced by the limbic system, especially the amygdala. Through the hypothalamus endocrine and anatomic responses can take place, suggesting that the hypothalamus provides the physiological connection between mental activity and physiological responses. Also the brainstem and thalamic activating systems are important structures in the development of an emotion since the arousal depends on the brainstem reticular formation and nonspecific thalamic nuclei.

The most often noted changes in personality are observed after damage to the frontal lobes. Most prominent changes are seen in cases of bilateral frontal damage. A characteristic feature of the frontal lobe syndrome is the lack of inhibition, impulsivity and lack of concern. Another characteristic feature is the mania for making puerile jokes (referred to as *Witzelsucht* in the classical German literature). Sometimes a tendency to repeat and perseverate is seen. A pathological passivity can be noted. In stark contrast, mutism is sometimes a sign of frontal lobe dysfunction, often associated with some degree of bradykinesia (i.e. a general slowness in movement and motor actions). According to Damasio (1979) it probably denotes bilateral mesial involvement of the frontal lobe. Goal-oriented behaviour is often impaired in patients with frontal lobe lesions. They are unable to manage the activities of daily life and they have great difficulties planning their near and long term future. The impaired integration of behaviour results in loss of capacity to think in abstract terms (Benton 1968).

Impairment of Inhibitory Control of Emotional Expression

Impairment of inhibitory control of emotional expression has been described by many authors (Taylor 1969; Bardach 1969; Espmark 1973). For instance, Benson (1973 and 1979) has described the **emotional lability** of pseudobulbar palsy as an *uninhibited emotional reaction to appropriate stimuli*. Pseudobulbar palsy requires bilateral upper motor neurone brain damage. The lability of emotion apparently represents an impairment of inhibitory control and should not be confused with post-stroke depression.

The impairment of emotional control should also be distinguished from emotional lability. In cases of loss of emotional control sudden crying (or rarely laughter) without adequate reason can occur (sometimes referred to as *pathological crying or laughing*). Other signs of pseudobulbar palsy are spastic dysarthria, dysphagia, increased primitive reflexes and urine incontinence. The emotional reactions that sometimes accompany pseudobulbar palsy are easily recognizable in the clinic. What we would normally consider as excessive emotional responses to relatively mild stimuli (e.g. a picture of a baby) are often observed. Dysarthria (flaccid) and dysphagia may

28

be present also in cases of brain stem pathology, but pathological crying is not found. The presence of emotional lability should not be considered as proof of pseudobulbar palsy, as it can occur in other conditions. A state of emotional lability can be seen in many patients with a sudden onset of a severe disease. It is accompanied by symptoms of fatigue, concentration problems, irritability, distractibility. The symptoms are most pronounced in the acute phase but may sometimes last for years.

Psychosocial Reactions in Aphasic Patients

Psychosocial reactions frequently seem to appear both among the aphasic patients themselves and their relatives. Psychosocial reactions refer to those aspects of behaviour which have interactional and social consequences. Biorn-Hansen (1957) listed five social areas where change took place among aphasic patients post onset:

alcohol intake increased;

there were role changes in the families;

their sexual habits changed;

they were overprotected;

patients became more dependent.

Friedman (1961) confirmed the altered social life and also pointed out the loneliness and loss of partners as important psychosocial events. Ullman (1962) confirmed the sexual changes and the altered social life. D'Afflitti & Weitz (1974) observed the overprotection as a common phenomenon in their unstructured patient-family groups. Ricco-Schwartz (1982) has also drawn attention to the negative effect on the children of aphasics as another important psychosocial consequence of aphasia. The tendency towards social isolation in aphasics was confirmed by Währborg and

Borenstein (1988) where it was significantly related to the spouses' rating of the physical handicap. It was shown that the worse the spouses rated their opinion about the physical impairment the more social isolation and the more lack of initiative was reported in the aphasics. No such connections were found between the degree of actual physical impairment as measured at the neurological examination and social isolation or lack of initiative. The results suggest that spouses' interpretation of the physical impairment is more important for the tendency towards social isolation than the actual degree of the physical impairment itself.

Unrealistic expectations and/or beliefs on the part of relatives regarding the significance and prognosis of the language impairment have been described (Friedman 1961; D'Afflitti & Weitz 1974; Taylor 1969). Oqvist *et al* (1982) reported that 50% of the aphasic patients in their group were unsatisfactorily informed about the handicap. Unrealistic expectations on recovery demonstrated in several studies may be a very important factor in therapy, since false beliefs may well be counter-productive in the struggle for recovery.

Other, more cognitive, impairments would appear to be associated with emotional and motivational aspects of recovery also. Impaired cognitive abilities such as difficulties in abstract thinking, abstract attitude and cognitive superficiality have been noted (Taylor 1969; Hurwitz & Adams 1972).

Summary

A remarkable variety and range of disturbances in emotional and psychosocial state have been reported in connection with brain damage and aphasia. These emotional and psychosocial problems do not occur exclusively with aphasia of course. Some appear closely related to the site, extent and nature of the brain damage (*primary* reactions) while others seem to be natural reactions to drastically changed life circumstances (*secondary* reactions). Some constellations of disturbance and developments in affective state are probably due to a combination of both primary and secondary causes. From a clinical perspective emotional and psychosocial factors may well have the effect of undermining much rehabilitation. However, for many of these problems useful intervention has been developed which can help to considerably improve the patients' situation and optimize possible gains from speech therapy.

Our current understanding suggests that the following appear to be important factors associated with the nature of an affective response to brain damage and aphasia:

1. The size and location of the brain injury appear to determine, at least in part, the initial nature of the disturbance.

2. A natural reactive depression can develop following brain damage.

3. The patient's perception of their own impairment has been demonstrated to influence the nature of their response to brain injury.

4. Family members perception of the impairment has been shown to influence psychosocial adjustment for both patient and relative.

5. Depressive state can increase with time since onset of brain injury.

Chapter 3

Aphasia and The Family

An area still often neglected in aphasia rehabilitation is the role of the family. As early as 1951, Wepman emphasized the importance of the family and friends in the rehabilitation process. A range of studies examining this question have confirmed the importance of those close to the aphasic person (Turnblom and Myers 1952; Biorn-Hansen 1957; Derman and Manaster 1967; Malone 1969; for review see Rollins 1987). In this chapter we examine the effects of aphasia on the family.

In the context of a group discussion programme involving the families of aphasic patients, Turnblom and Myers (1952) found that responses by family members to their situation included pity, shame and guilt. They pointed out that the problems faced by the family might be reflected in the aphasic person's response to rehabilitation, affecting both outlook and motivation. In an anecdotal study Biorn-Hansen (1957) suggested that the level of family support has a major effect on the patient's response to therapy, although no empirical data was given to support this view. According to Biorn-Hansen the most common problem faced by the family members he studied was the changes in role necessitated by the illness.

In an informal, explorative study based on unstructured interviews with 25 people who represented the families of 20 aphasic patients, Malone (1969) identified nine problems reported by family members: role changes, irritability, guilt feelings, altered social life, financial problems, job neglect, health problems, over-solicitousness, rejection and the effect on children. An empirical study of the attitudes expressed by the families of aphasic individuals (Malone, Ptacek and Malone 1970) identified retributive guilt, unrealistic attitudes, rejection, overprotection and social withdrawal in the family members.

In the late 1970's comparative studies of psychosocial readjustment in the spouses of aphasic patients began to appear (Kinsella and Duffy 1978, 1979). The major findings in these studies confirmed earlier less objective observations that spouses of aphasic individuals experienced a higher incidence of problems and adjustment difficulties than the spouses of non-aphasic stroke patients. The areas that were particularly impaired were social and leisure activities and marital relationships. Aphasia appeared to be particularly disruptive in that the marriages were characterized by problems of interpersonal communication, diminished sexual satisfaction and loss of partnership. An increased incidence of minor psychiatric disorders was found amongst all spouses of stroke patients but this was more pronounced in the spouses of aphasic subjects. Interestingly, wives of aphasic patients revealed a significantly greater incidence of minor psychiatric disorders than wives of non-aphasic stroke patients.

In 1983 *The Code-Müller Protocols* were introduced (also called Code-Müller Scales), a short questionnaire used to elicit perceptions of psychosocial adjustment from patients, family members and professionals (Müller and Code 1983; Müller, Code and Mugford 1983; Herrmann and Wallesch 1990; Code and Müller In Preparation). Findings include an incongruity of perceptions between spouses, therapists and patients. Spouses and other family members were found to be more optimistic about psychosocial adjustment than speech therapists, who were the most pessimistic. This could be interpreted in the light of the findings of Malone *et al* (1979) as an expression of unrealistic attitudes on the part of the family members although it may have been that the therapists had a less than complete knowledge of how the aphasic individuals manage outside the clinic (cf Holland 1977). These incongruities between different groups may reflect role positions or attitudes: family members may feel they have little alternative but to express optimism and therapists the opposite.

A few studies have found that the presence of aphasia in one partner can lead to a feeling of marital dissatisfaction in the other (Kinsella and Duffy 1979; Williams and Freer 1986). Williams and Freer's spouses completed a *Knowledge of Aphasia* questionnaire and pre- and post-stroke forms of a *Marital Satisfaction Scale* (MSS). Although there was a significant negative change between the pre- and post-stroke MSS scores, indicating reduced marital satisfaction, neither the spouses' knowledge of aphasia, nor the severity of aphasia was related to their marital satisfaction. It was also found that spouses of mildly impaired patients had less knowledge about aphasia than did those of severely impaired patients. A somewhat surprising finding emerged from Währborg and Borenstein (1988) which aimed to identify the psychosocial problems experienced by spouses. While the spouses reported a decreased sexual interest they denied any other change in emotions or behaviour. The possibility of the spouses' reports being *idealized* was strongly considered, but it is still surprising that they did not actually report any further problems.

Spouses' Understanding of The Communication Problems of Their Partner

A number of studies have drawn attention to the level and quality of information given to stroke patients and their relatives (Artes 1967; Haese 1970; Overs and Healy 1970) and generally conclude from their interviews with the patients and their families that they are not given sufficient information about the stroke and its effects.

The issue of spouses' understanding of the communication disabilities of their aphasic partner is a crucial one to rehabilitation and it will influence the quality of communication in the family. The problems faced by family members in adaptation to a new communication situation means that the family members exercise an important influence on rehabilitation. The spouses' verbal behaviour, coloured by their understanding of their partner's communication difficulties, can either facilitate or impede language recovery, as suggested by Helmick *et al* (1976). The main approach to gaining information on spouses understanding of the communication difficulties of their spouses, has been to examine how they judge their partners' language ability and to contrast this with performance on standardised clinical aphasia tests.

Helmick *et al* (1976) compared performance on the Porch Index of Communicative Ability (PICA) with the judgements made by the spouses of their partner's communicative abilities. The Overall PICA score was taken as a measure of each aphasic patient's language skills. The Functional Communication Profile (FCP) (Taylor 1965) was used to measure each spouse's understanding of their aphasic partner's communication. The speech pathologist who had diagnosed the individual aphasic patient independently completed the FCP for the patient. Results showed that the spouses tended to assign higher FCP scores to their partners than did the speech pathologists. The speech pathologist's FCP scores seemed to be more comparable with the PICA scores. The authors conclude that the spouses tended to view their aphasic partner's communication as less impaired than it actually was. The authors suggest that this could mean that the spouses are providing some emotional or moral support for their partner. Assuming that it is the spouses who have the more unrealistic perceptions, then this may lead to the establishment of unrealistic expectations for language performance and to the use of inappropriate amounts and types of language while interacting with their communicatively impaired partner.

Discussing this study, Holland (1977) pointed out the difficulties involved in drawing these conclusions. She argued that the spouse is in a better position to make use of contextual cues and might therefore be more accurate in assessing the communicative ability of the aphasic patient. Helmick *et al* (1977) in their reply to Holland claimed that the data does indicated a discrepancy between the evaluation of language skills made by spouses and therapists.

Support for this fundamental finding comes from Flowers *et al* (1979) who investigated how well the performance of 20 aphasic persons on a language test was predicted by family members or others who were in frequent contact with the aphasic person. Family members tended to overestimate the communicative abilities of the aphasic individuals. Careful reading of this report reveals that the spouses were able to correctly predict the item-by-item test outcome in 71% of the items and failed to predict the outcome in 29% of the cases. Seventy-two per cent of the inaccurate predictions (the 29%) were overestimations of performance.

In 1988 our group in Gothenburg (Hedberg-Borenstein *et al* 1988) carried out a study involving 15 consecutive referrals to the department who suffered from aphasia due to a CVA during the period June 28, 1984 - May 20, 1986. All patients were married or were living together with another adult and all were native speakers of Swedish. The time since onset was 1 to 3 years and no signs of dementia were present. The median age of the eleven aphasics who remained in the study (seven men and four women) was 54 years and the median time since onset was 26 months. The median duration of marriage was 30 years. Seven subjects were diagnosed as mixed syndromes, one as aphasia with very mild anomia, one transcortical motor aphasia and two with conduction aphasia.

Spouses were interviewed before the aphasic subjects were tested to avoid the spouse being influenced by the actual outcome on the aphasia test. The spouse and the aphasic, respectively, had to rate on a Visual Analogue Scale (see Figure 3) the

Figure 3: An example of a Visual Analogue Scale (VAS) item.

Do You Ever Feel Sad?

NEVER ——————————————————————— **ALWAYS**

ability of their aphasic partner in the following areas: auditory comprehension, repetition of words and sentences, naming, reading aloud, reading comprehension, writing and finally the overall severity of aphasia. Note that we did not ask either spouse or patient to predict performance on the aphasia test, but rather to rate different aspects of language ability. Each visual analogue scale was an 100 mm long line drawn on a card and the patient and spouse had to rate the degree of ability from *absent* (0 mm) to *excellent* (100 mm) by dissecting the line at any point between these two poles. An important feature of this simple but sensitive technique is that there is no learning effect, and measures can be taken at any time without previous self-ratings affecting subsequent ones. Each patient was then tested with Reinvang's aphasia battery (Reinvang and Engvik 1980), a standardized Swedish variant of the Boston Aphasia Examination (Goodglass and Kaplan 1972).

Table 1: Correlations between aphasia test outcome and the capacity of aphasics and their spouses to judge linguistic ability.

	Auditory Comp.	Repetition	Naming	Reading	Reading Aloud	Writing Comp.	Sum	Severity
Aphasics vs Spouses	0.6707*	0.22903	0.47032	0.61319*	0.70932*	0.40909	0.53303	0.79271**
Aphasics vs Test	0.41126	0.33951	0.15705	0.42697	0.44734	0.39728	0.45558	0.27652
Spouses vs Test	0.46779	0.28134	0.61153*	0.79622**	0.64972*	0.37418	0.42727	0.47809

The Spearman Correlation Coefficients are shown in the table (* $p < 0.05$, ** $p < 0.01$)

Table 1 presents the main findings from this study. Comparisons are listed to the left of the table. Firstly, (first row) the patients predictions were compared to the spouses and there was congruity between them for auditory and reading comprehension, for reading aloud and for overall severity. For these areas at least, there was evidence of significant agreement between the groups. In the second row the test performance was compared to the predictions of the aphasic patients where little evidence is available for agreement. Patients felt their language impairments not as bad as the aphasia test suggests. Finally, in the third row the outcome on the test was compared to the predictions of the spouses. Significant correlations for naming, reading aloud and reading comprehension were found. While there was significant agreement between patients and spouses on severity of language impairment (first row), both groups (second and third rows) judged the impairment to be less severe than the Aphasia Quotient (the sum of the subtests in Reinvang's test) would suggest.

The findings of previous studies, that spouses tend to overestimate the ability of the aphasics could not be verified in our study. On the contrary, both patients and spouses seemed to underestimate severity. The Functional Communication Profile, used by Helmick *et al* (1976) in their study, is more a measure of the functional communication abilities of the individual, while the aphasia test battery measures more general linguistic impairments. For patients and spouses, actual functional performance is conceivably of more importance to them both.

In the study by Flowers *et al* (1979) the spouses had to predict the outcome of each sub-test item, not estimate language ability. Such a task would appear to be more difficult and therefore is more liable to mistakes than our approach. Despite this, most of the predictions by spouses reported by Flowers *et al (1979)* were correct. The aphasics and their spouses estimated the overall severity of the aphasia as much more pronounced than would be concluded from the Aphasia Quotient. Bearing our own results in mind, this suggests that the aphasics and their spouses considered more than the linguistic aspects in their ratings of severity of the aphasia.

Conclusions

Despite the variability in the approaches in many studies, most of the research points in the same direction. Members of *aphasic families* can have considerable and significant difficulties which can arise as a result of one member having aphasia. There seem to be three areas were problems and obstacles to rehabilitation occur:

Aphasia and the Family

1) family members seem to be particularly prone to developing minor psychiatric disorders (anxiety reactions, guilt feelings, irritability, agitation, etc.) themselves;

2) the nature and the quality of interaction between the spouse and the aphasic partner tends to change, leading to reductions in social and sex life;

3) there is an apparent lack of knowledge about the handicap on the part of family members and this lack of knowledge might be a source of misunderstandings and cause the harbouring of unrealistic beliefs.

Mulhall (1978) who investigated the mutual influence aphasic stroke patients and their relatives have on each other, even suggests that the spouse's reaction to the communication disorder aggravates the verbal output of the patient.

However, despite our improved understanding of these difficulties counselling and therapy are seldom offered to such families in the normal course of clinical practice. Family therapy is a special kind of psychotherapy and we discuss its application in detail in Chapter 6.

Chapter 4

Towards a Model of Psychological Reactions to Brain Damage and Aphasia

The previous chapters have concentrated on the results of brain damage and *what* happens in the lives of aphasic individuals. In this chapter the focus will be on *why* changes occur, on the mechanisms underlying the different changes that appear in aphasics as well as in their families. This is of major relevance for diagnostics and therapeutics.

When Reitan and Davidson (1974) tried to state the role of the neuropsychologist they wrote:

> *The clinical neuropsychologist is not merely interested in differentiating brain damage from other diagnostic possibilities; he is also interested in making refined descriptions of clinical conditions including inferences as to location and extent of brain damage, if any, and probable medical and psychological conditions accounting for the abnormal behaviour. Increasingly, he is interested in prognosis of recovery, rehabilitation potentials, and management alternatives for the patient* (p.3).

Under *neuropsychologist* we can include *aphasiologist* and *aphasia therapist*.

In order to discuss the reactions to brain damage and aphasia, a theory of the relationships between brain, emotions and behaviour is required. In this chapter some important features of such a theory will be outlined.

Towards a Model of Psychosocial Reactions

The Development of Self

> *Becoming a fully human being depends on a maturation process in*
> *which the acquisition of speech plays an enormous part. One learns*
> *not only to perceive, and to interpret one's perceptions, but also to be*
> *a person, and to be a self* (Popper 1977: p. 47).

The Self is basically a social self since a self without a social context is unthinkable. The brain could be seen as the bearer of the self - the biological representation of the self's existence. Two parallel systems can be identified as a consequence of this view: a **representational** self, where we perceive, identify and experience the world, which is dependent upon the **physical** world. Both the representational and physical systems can be appreciated as hierarchically organized. We can see the representational system as the psychological and social self and the physical system as the biological self.

The Representational System

Representation of the outer world is a necessary activity of the central nervous system, and, in fact, the normal functioning of the brain depends on constantly changing stimulation. This ongoing activity in the representational system acts as a continuing arousal reaction in the neo-cortex which maintains mental awareness.

The final representation, our mental map of the world, is therefore dependent on our senses. The actual experience of self - the *empirical* self - is developed through a progressively ongoing interaction between our self and the external world. The social self requires relationships to develop (Cooley 1902, Mead 1934). In extreme isolation - like in the shocking case where a mother kept her infant daughters in solitude in secluded rooms over a period of years, giving them just enough attention to keep them alive - humans tend to have problems in developing a sense of self (Davis 1947). In this case the 2 children were discovered around age 6 years. Both were severely mentally retarded, they exhibited behaviour resembling that of infancy, they could not talk and one of them could not even walk. They exhibited fear of strangers and appeared unable to form relationships with other persons.

Experiences from laboratory experiments (for an overview see Zubek 1974) indicates that interaction produces vital stimulation for the brain to uphold higher cortical or mental functions. It has been reported that social isolation causes retardation (Davis 1947) and it has been shown that sensory deprivation speeds up the degenerative changes normally associated with ageing and enhances the loss of functional cells in the central nervous system (Oster 1976).

Perception is an absolute requirement for building up a representation of the world and the perception of relationships, our deep understanding of the nature and worth of relationships, is the fundamental basis for development of the self. *Empirical self* can be seen as the second step in the development of self and can be defined as the person's own perception and appreciation of their self.

Interaction and Relationships

It is often said that *man is a social animal*, and socialization is an integral element in the nature of humanity. Interaction between two human beings constitutes a relationship and relationships are built up in a hierarchical manner. The initial relationship experienced by the infant has the character of a symbiosis, *I am a part of my mother*. The infant's empirical self is strictly limited during the first six months of living, but already during the first year of life the infant develops toward separation and individualization. During the third year the child has reached a point where it experiences a certain degree of constancy in the world. The world is no longer a series of snap-shots, but exists; even when the child shuts it's eyes. The interactional development is primarily due to the relationships developed in play and games. The child learns to decentre from itself to the possible worlds of others, take the position of the other, through the games. Mead suggested some time ago (Mead 1934) that this outer organized community or social group, which gives to the individual a unity of self, could be called *the generalized other*. Thus, in order to develop the relationship to one's self (empirical self) the child has to develop relationships with others.

One's relationship to one's self is most probably unique and species-specific; humans being the only mammals who enjoy such an experience. Introspection is exclusively human, and is a function of the organization of our central nervous system. As a consequence of this exclusive ability the human seems to be the most egocentric animal on earth, but also the only species with a mental representation of death. We all know that we are going to die and this fundamental realization may engender the basic need for a God, an explanation to the meaning of life and death.

In play and games children discover the other human beings surrounding them and the generalized other becomes a part of the social self, thereby supporting the internalization of social norms and attitudes. However, this process does not take place in an environmental vacuum. The child who becomes an adolescent has incorporated cognitive and perceptual structures which are tied to emotions in the same manner as the social development of the self. As Popper (1977) pointed out, the acquisition of speech has a tremendous influence on this process. But apart from the importance of perceptions and language in the empirical self, human beings also have "perceptions" and "language" for another self - a phenomena often called *projection*; i.e., the transfer of my own perceptions to another person or target (a dog for instance).

So far it has been hypothesized that humans have significant relationships with themselves as well as with others. However, another important dimension of relationship takes place in everyday life, the relationship to objects. Objects are inanimate things like furniture, rings, cars or even memories. These *things* do not represent the self but offer the individual targets for projection. We endow an object with a soul and through this process the object becomes animate. The existence of this animation (giving inanimate things a self) appears to be a basic need for human beings to relate themselves to the physical world, where the existence of other things is the manifest proof of the self's existence.

In every day life the forming of "relationships" to objects is common. Many people name their cars and their boats. Some people even talk to their potted plants. Apparently these relationships are obvious and recognizable in elderly and brain damaged people. When an old woman is moved from her own house to an institution a basic security in her self is taken away from her - her familiar relationships to objects in the physical world that surrounded her. This world is not exchangeable since she has developed an interaction with the things in her house, with the house itself, the rooms, the furniture and so on. These things and the relationships with them are parts of her self. To move her is therefore a threat to her self, especially since it is more difficult to adapt to new relationships for elderly and brain damaged persons. A single object can act in a human life as an anchor for the empirical self, it might be that dogs or other pets often play this role in peoples' lives. Such a model of the self is at variance with many modern approaches to caring for elderly and brain damaged people, which tend to emphasize removing the individual from their familiar surroundings. Such circumstances can hasten and exacerbate the decline of self.

The next dimension of interaction seems to develop much later in life. As pointed out the child develops constancy in the belief of the existence of others, the existence of their own mind and in their relationship to external objects; but the fourth dimension is a need which grows out of maturation and new fundamental questions arise about life. At a certain point in human life questions arise that cannot be answered at the existing three levels of interaction. Questions of a fundamentally philosophical nature like *Who am I?*, *What is the meaning of my life?* etc., can be understood from a representational point of view as the search for a God or a universal power. From an interactionist point of view the development of a meta self, the God, is a transcendence of the Self and would be impossible without former socialization.

To summarize this section, four levels of interaction can be described:

    a) interaction with one's self;

    b) interaction with others;

    c) interaction with objects and;

    4. interaction with a god.

These interactions or relationships play a significant role in the development of the self and are therefore crucial in human development and life.

Relationships are Communication

Interactions between people are, by definition, exchanges of behaviours. Nothing needs to be known about the motives, the emotions or otherwise implicit aspects of the exchange to observe the behaviours. Communication is also implicitly part of such behavioural exchanges; there is no such state as *no communication*. An interaction or a relationship requires communication, otherwise no interaction will take place. In this sense relationships are communication.

Communication can be expressed in a variety of manners, of course, but the technical aspects of communication will not be dealt with here. For the purposes of this book we should note that aphasia, as an impairment of communication, interferes with the ability to maintain relationships in a very sudden and dramatic way.

The Physical System

As pointed out earlier the physical system is the biological representation of emotions and the self. The living organism is in no way a static system but is always in a state of constant activity. This activity characterizes the single individual as well as the species in general. The development of emotions as well as the self tends to be governed by this evolutionary fact. The physiological basis of emotions has been briefly discussed in Chapter 2. It will be discussed here only in the context of its principal relationship to the development of the self.

It has been shown that emotions depend on activity of several anatomic structures: the cerebral cortex, limbic structures, hypothalamus and the brain stem. The internal processing among and between these structures have been interpreted differently. An interesting interpretation is made by Jason Brown (1988) who has developed the *microgenic theory* of brain function. The microgenic process deals with evolutionary facts:

> *An organism is active in the present. The ontogenesis of the organism is a record in the experience of living things; its phylogenesis, a theory about a period before the living record. We accept that maturation goes into the shaping of a particular stage in behaviour, and that ontogenic form has an evolutionary background* (Brown 1988: p. 6).

Brown describes the hierarchical microgenic structure as follows:

> *The microgenic process is hierarchial; later levels differentiate out of earlier ones. The series of levels leading from the inception of a mental state to the final representation forms a complex structure. Mind does not appear at the surface of this structure but obtains at each moment*

in a series of emergent states. The complete structure - the series of unfolding stages, not their outcome, the representation - is the neuropsychological correlate of a cognitive state. The representation incorporates into its structure, and is part of, the whole hierarchic series which precedes it. In other words, processing stages that underlie or are submerged within a performance constitute part of the structure of that performance, just as stages of development in childhood persist as the subconscious motives or the experiential context guiding the cognition of the adult (Brown 1988: p. 7).

So, according to microgenic theory almost any site of brain damage will be important for the understanding of the final emotional and behavioural outcome. However, through experience we know that certain lesions with certain locations can be more important for emotional and behavioural outcome than others. Disturbances in motivational behaviour tend to be more related to lesions in the limbic system and perceptual disturbances are more frequent in posterior lesions, etc. These different observations could be understood within a framework of systems theory (Bertalanffy 1968). Even though a certain area of the brain is directly connected to a specific behaviour *any* damage might interfere with the functions primarily represented in other parts of the brain (cf diaschisis phenomena).

Another hypothesis used to explain the outcome of physical damage to the brain is the principle of *mass action*, associated with Karl Lashley (1929). If the brain loses mass, as for instance in the degenerative process of Altzeimer's disease, there is no focal lesion to explain the behavioural changes, but the brain will lose in its total capabililities to express emotions and behaviours.

Aphasia and Mental Changes

In acquired aphasia two obvious facts are present: there is a sudden onset of brain damage and there is a similar sudden disturbance in communicative ability. The brain damage interferes with neural activities which result in loss of neural functioning in some cases characterized by *interruption* (e.g. loss of inhibitory control of emotions) and some cases *destruction* of primary centres in motivational behaviour (e.g. reduction in motivational behaviour resulting in apathy, dysphoria). The brain damage also causes a *depletion* in biochemical activity in the neurons (e.g. causing depression, anxiety or other disorders).

The central feature of the aphasic state is of course the sudden onset of a communicative disability that accounts for a sudden interruption in relational life, since relationships cannot exist without communication. This interruption has an immediate impact on how individual's perceive themselves and their self. According to what has been claimed earlier, this sudden but persistent change will influence all relational aspects of the individual. The reduced ability to cope and the threat to the self act as signals to develop stress-reactions and minor psychiatric disorders.

As we have seen, mental changes in aphasic individuals can be either a result of the brain damage *per se*, due to the onset of a communicative disability, or both. Many of the reported disorders observed with aphasia (see Chapter 2) are most likely not directly related to the aphasic state itself. With the theoretical framework outlined in this chapter, the clinician may find it easier to sort out the disorders linked to the aphasic state and thereby be in a better position to offer appropriate treatment.

Chapter 5

The Assessment of Emotional and Psychosocial Disorder in Aphasic Individuals and Their Families

In this essentially clinically oriented and practical chapter instruments and techniques are discussed which will help the clinician to identify and evaluate important emotional and psychosocial disorders in the aphasic person and in the aphasic family. At the beginning of a chapter like this it is necessary to stress the importance of correct identification or diagnosis. Though few studies have yet been completed, the available evidence confirms that we have reason to believe that mental obstacles are counter productive in the rehabilitation of aphasia, and this is probably true for both psychosocial and linguistic rehabilitation. Many of the complicating psychic and social disorders appearing in aphasic patients and their families are problems that can be dealt with successfully. We are confident that problems observed have different etiologies and, therefore, most probably require different therapeutic approaches. Without a correct diagnosis, therefore, we will continue to grope in the dark and the patients and their families will continue to suffer from therapeutic neglect. We look at family diagnosis later in the chapter, but begin with assessment of the aphasic individual.

General Aims of Evaluation

The following general principles are useful for the systematic evaluation of the patient's problem:

1. The first aim of the diagnostic procedure is to *describe* the problem and to possibly outline its *etiology*. The description of the problem should represent a) the patient's view, b) the spouse's view, and c) the examiner's observations. The etiologic diagnosis aims at crystallizing the *determinants* of the present reaction or disorder. The determinants can be a) intrapersonal, which include premorbid personality and self-perception, age and psychiatric history, b) interpersonal, which includes family, friends and other significant persons, c) pathology-related, which includes representational as well as physical aspects and/or d) sociocultural and economic, which influence values, beliefs and attitudes to the present state. This stage of evaluation can be called the *qualitative* stage.

2. The second aim is to *quantify* the problem, that is, to judge the severity of the problem. We can call this the *quantitative* stage.

3. The third aim in the diagnostic procedure is to *interpret* obtained data. This interpretation serves as the examiner's working hypothesis of the nature of the problem. This stage we can call the *operational* stage.

4. A fourth and important aspect of the evaluative procedure is to give hope and comfort to the patient. An important message to impart to the patient is therefore one of sincerity and empathy.

The Examination

The Interview

To interview an aphasic person is of course challenging in itself, but most speech pathologists, psychologists and physicians working with brain damaged individual's are familiar with the difficulties involved. It might be unnecessary, therefore, to remind the reader that an interview of this kind takes time. One should also remember to let the patient take *their* time. The quality of the interview will increase considerably if the patient has the feeling that the examiner wants to understand his or her problems. In order to get as broad a picture as possible of the presenting problems it is worth while gathering information from as many people familiar with the patient's situation as possible. It is recommended that the patient should decide whether or not they want their spouse to be involved in the interview. To involve the spouse as well requires more skill on the part of the examiner. Sometimes it is a good idea to first interview the aphasic person and then the spouse.

The interview should cover the following six important issues, however not necessarily in this order since the interview has to be structured according to the situation:

1. Description of the presenting problems. What is bothering the patient and in what way? What is most difficult in life at the moment apart from the aphasic condition? Is there anything the patient wants to change in his or her life (apart from the aphasia of course)?

2. Premorbid personality. Have there been changes in personality and self-esteem? Has the patient changed in mood since onset of the aphasia, and if so, in what way? What kind of emotional or psychological problems did the patient have before onset, if any?

3. Time since onset of a) the brain damage and the aphasia, and b) the presenting problems. How was the initial discovery of being aphasic experienced? Has the experience of the aphasic state changed? What

is the patient's opinion about the relationship of the present problems to the aphasic state?

4. Duration of the present problems.

5. Knowledge about the handicap. How much has the patient been informed about her/his handicap? How much has the family been informed? Are there present any unrealistic beliefs on the nature of the condition?

6. Sociocultural changes. In what ways has the patient's social life altered since onset of aphasia? Is there a tendency towards social isolation?

Systematic Observations

The quality of the observations made by the examiner constitute a powerful tool in the evaluation of the patient's psychic and social status. One of the most important clinical skills is the ability to systematically observe and to draw conclusions from these observations. It may be worth recalling Sherlock Holmes' perpetually repeated statement to Dr Watson, *It is a matter of training Watson*. The following suggestions are useful aids in systematically structuring observation.

In 1974 Lipowski put forward a *law* for discussing the personal meaning of illness: *A patient's overall response to illness and disability and his motivation to get well, are related to the subjectively experienced losses and/or gains derived from the illness.* According to Lipowski, three distinct patterns of coping styles can be identified which follow from this law:

Assessment

1. *Tackling*. This is the adoption of an active attitude to illness where *fighting* is the order of the day. Therapeutic alliance is assured, for the patient wishes to be rid of his or her problems as soon as possible.

2. *Capitulation*. This is the adoption of a passive or dependent attitude. Cooperation is poor and excessive demands for support are made with little or no attempt to achieve independence.

3. *Avoiding*. This is shown by those who cannot accept their handicap or treatment and is therefore characterized by considerable denial.

Certain behavioural symptoms are more common in aphasic patients and should therefore be looked out for. As observed above, an important aspect of behaviour is *activity*. Overactivity can be expressed as a marked restlessness and overactivity of bodily movements often involving the larger joints are common. This restlessness is often seen in euphoric and manic states. A decreased activity might be an expression of psycho-motor retardation seen in depressive states. Decreased activity is often overlooked in hospitals since this behaviour is more convenient and therefore attracts little attention. The degree of *co-operation* on the part of the patient is another important aspect of the behaviour analysis. A common reaction observed in aphasic patients is negativism, a refusal or active resistance to do what is suggested.

Language expresses more than linguistic and intellectual messages. Speech and voice also reflect emotional state. Changes in speech and voice, in addition to aphasia or dysarthria, can indicate changes in psychic state. Very slow speech or voice low in amplitude or monotonic can sometimes be related to a depressive state. Speech contaminated with rhymes, puns and sometimes clang associations such as *ding-dong-King-Kong* indicates an indifference often associated with right hemisphere damage. Also associated with right hemisphere damage are disturbances in emotional tone or affective language (Code 1987). In some cases affective language will be under- and in some, overemphasized. Affective disorders are common among aphasics and it is therefore important to observe the patients' affective behaviour.

The range of emotional and psychological reactions observed in brain damage are described in detail in earlier Chapters (2-4). We will mention only the main features of behaviour to look out for. In depressive patients sadness, hopelessness and irritability will be found; but even just guilt feelings and feelings of worthlessness are common. The opposite emotion, euphoria, is found in some cases but it is not as common as the depressive reaction. Emotional lability, as previously discussed, is the rapid change in emotional tone to tears or laughter with slight or even no emotional provocation. This lability is a common feature in many cases of brain damage. Feelings of shame, guilt, irritability, etc., have been described in aphasic patients, but could of course be found in any person with or without a handicap. Regression, a tendency to behave childish, is sometimes found in aphasia, but most often in combination with dementia. Denial and rejection as well as projection are other defense mechanisms often observed in aphasic patients (see Chapter 2).

Disturbances of *thought processes and content* are observed in aphasic patients. Whether these disturbances are the result of the brain damage or a secondary psychic reaction has not been explored to a satisfactory extent. A range of disturbances can be recognized and noted. Common features of brain damaged are difficulties in concentration and attention, also the inability to simultaneously do more than one thing at a time. If the radio is on in the room or someone else is talking the aphasic person often fails to concentrate on the topic of conversation. Delusions of persecution and sin are sometimes seen in depressed patients. In some cases ideas of unreality or derealization might be found. Perceptional disorders are occasionally due to the psychic state rather than a result of the brain damage. Hallucinations occasionally occur, and should be noted.

In summary, all observations made by the examiner might be of importance for adequate diagnosis and treatment.   No matter how sophisticated our formal assessment techniques, or biochemical or other techniques, nothing compensates for careful clinical observation.

The Physical Examination

As well as the normal routine medical examination, the physical examination should also include a full neurological status examination where the patient's difficulties can be related to localisation of damage.   Observations of the patients general reactions and posture, facial expression, co-operativeness, eyes, reactions to verbal instructions, muscular tonus and emotional reactivity should be noted during the examination.

In most cases the investigation of psychological and social consequences of aphasia is carried out by speech pathologists, psychologists and others who are not medically trained.   In some cases the patient may not have had a medical examination and it is an advantage to refer the patient to a doctor, preferably a neurologist, for a full medical examination.   Inpatients most usually have already had a physical examination but it is suggested that the clinician takes full interest in any implications of the results of this physical examination.

Biochemical Data

In recent years considerable progress has been made in identifying the various transmitter substances in the brain. The distribution of these transmitter substances has been mapped out and the molecular events of synaptic transmission have been clarified. These diverse chemical transmitters act as biochemical signals between the neurons. The transmitters are not randomly distributed throughout the brain but are localized in specific clusters of neurons whose axons project to other highly specific brain regions. Some 30 different substances are known or believed to be transmitters in the brain. Also the variety of different mechanisms by which the transmitters exert their effects are becoming apparent. Each transmitter acts in an excitatory or inhibitory fashion on neurons but they can also, instead of directly exciting or inhibiting a target neuron, act presynaptically on an adjacent nerve terminal to increase or decrease the release of transmitter from that nerve terminal.

The transmitters are particularly important in the context of depression after brain damage. The cause of post-stroke depression has been suggested to be connected with an interruption in cathecolaminergic (norepinephrine and epinephrine) pathways, thereby causing a profound drop in brain norepinephrine levels. Left anterior lesions interrupt more such pathways than posterior lesions do (Robinson and Szetala 1981). This hypothesis, designated the *catecholamine hypothesis of affective disorder*, proposes that some, if not all, depressions are associated with an absolute or relative deficiency of catecholamines, particularly norepinephrine (NA), at functionally important receptor sites in the brain (Schildkraut 1965). Apart from catecholamine and norepinephrine, other transmitters have been found to be important in the development of depression. Dopamine (DA) and 5-hydroxytryptamine have been found closely aligned to the melancholic syndrome (Baldessarini 1975). Whereas the etiology of depression remains to be established the altered functions in monoaminergic systems calls for attention. It has been found that drugs increasing the levels of monoamines in the brain are effective in the treatment of depression.

The metabolites of the transmitters described above can be measured in biological fluids (blood, urine and cerebrospinal fluid). Sophisticated and reliable techniques have been developed to examine the metabolites in cerebrospinal fluid (Svennerholm 1989). The measure of 5-hydroxytryptamine metabolites (5-HIAA) and norepinephrine metabolites (HMPG) are important steps in the diagnosis of depression since a low proportion of these metabolites are considered characteristic of *biological* depressions (Maas 1975; Agren 1980) and post-stroke depressions (Robinson and Szetala 1981;

Währborg and Borenstein 1988). Dysfunction in neuroendocrine regulation has been found in depressed subjects (Carroll *et al* 1976 a,b).

For different reasons it is important to distinguish melancholia from other depressions and psychiatric disorders. A specific laboratory test for the diagnosis of melancholia has been developed to facilitate this distinction (Carroll *et al* 1981). The test is based on one of the observed neuroendocrine dysfunctions, namely the failure to suppress serum cortisol following dexamethasone administration (a synthetic cortisol). This failure has also been observed in aphasic patients with a major post-stroke depression (Lipsey *et al*. 1985: Reding *et al*. 1985).

The technique used to examine this failure, the dexamethasone suppression test (DST) (Carroll *et al*. 1981), is simple to adopt. The overnight DST procedure is the most common. One milligram of oral dexamethasone is given at 11:00 PM on day one. Blood samples for plasma cortisol determination are obtained at 8:00 AM, 4:00 PM and 11:00 PM the following day. The cortisol measures can be done by competitive protein binding assay or radioimmunoassay. The test should be considered positive if the 4:00 PM or the 11:00 cortisol level are more than 5 ug/dl for competitive protein binding assay or more than 6,4 ug/dl for radioimmunoassay technique. The sensitivity and the specificity varies with the criterion values used. Carroll *et al* (1981) reported an overall sensitivity ranging from 39 (plasma cortisol criterion value of 6 ug/dl) to 53 per cent (criterion value of 3 ug/dl). The overall specificity ranged from 85 (criterion value of 3 ug/dl) to 97 per cent (criterion value of 6 ug/dl). The technique has proved valuable in the diagnosis of major post-stroke depression and is therefore, together with analysis of monoaminemetabolites, an important medical contribution in the diagnosis of depression in aphasics.

Psychological Tests, Scales, and Questionnaires

The methodological problems in emotional and psychosocial work in aphasia are the same from a scientific and clinical perspective. One of the most important variables in clinical examinations is the clinician or examiner him or herself, and this bias is most often not considered in clinical or scientific reports. If the clinical examination involves tests, scales, questionnaires or other empirical tools, even more opportunity is given the clinician to influence results since the answers from the aphasic patient are influenced by the way instructions are given and checked out. Another bias in clinical examination involving different tests is the obvious fact that most tests, scales or questionnaires are not designed specifically for aphasic individuals.

Conventionally, four fundamental psychometric criteria should be borne in mind when evaluating a clinical test or rating scale for clinical use:

> 1. *Standardization* concerns two things: a) where the procedure, apparatus and scoring have been fixed, or standardised, so that precisely the same test can be given at different times and places by different testers and none of these variables should influence the results of the test; b) the test has been standardised on a group of *normal* subjects matched for any important variables such as age, sex, educational level, etc., so that performance by a patient can be compared to a *normal* performance and interpreted in the light of normal performance.

> 2. The *validity* of a test may be defined as the extent to which differences in scores on it reflect true differences among individuals, groups, or situations in the characteristic which it seeks to measure, or true differences in the same individual, group, or situation from one occasion to another, rather than constant or random errors. The test should be a valid assessment of the thing it seeks to assess. There are different types of validity. *Predictive validity* answers the question, does

the test score predict a certain future performance? *Content validity* concerns whether the test gives a fair measure of performance on a set of tasks and is used to compare the individual test items logically to each other. *Construct validity* concerns the extent to which the scores can be described theoretically.

3. *Reliability* refers to whether the measurement procedure, and variations in scores is due to inconsistencies in measurement. A test should have good inter-judge reliability (testers should score or rate behaviours similarly). Test-retest reliability concerns whether the test produces a similar performance by a testee each time it is administered. In the ideal situation the measurement should be free from random or variable errors.

Rating Scales

Rating scales are commonly used in clinical assessment and clinical research. Here the tester can rate a performance or behaviour by a patient, usually on a 3, 5 or 7 point scale and a large number have been devised over the years. Some of them have been developed for exclusive purposes and others for more general use in psychological and social contexts. It is of course impossible to cover all the scales that might be of interest for the aphasiologist. The following selection are the most common assessment scales in research and clinical contexts and those which fulfil at least elementary requirements on scientific standards.

The Visual Analogue Scale (VAS).
We discussed the VAS in Chapter 3. The origin of this simple but widely used scale is uncertain, but it was introduced as a measurement for feelings by Aitken (1969).

Usually, the VAS consists of a 100 mm long line printed on a card (illustrated in Figure 3, Chapter 3: p. 36). It is a self-rating scale based on semantic differentials where the subject is asked to rate his or her attitude in relation to two extremes poles where one end represents a rating of 0% and the other 100%. Measuring the distance from one end of the scale to the subject's mark gives a numerical rating.

The technique is simple to understand and very sensitive to small variations because of it's construction. The scale is also easy to work with statistically. Even hemiplegic and severely aphasic patients are usually able to understand and respond to simple questions used in visual analogue scales. The technique offers a simple way of measuring attitudes even in aphasics, and the scale can be used as often as desired as there is no learning effect.

Depression Scales

The most widely used and reliable scales for the assessment of depression are the Zung Self Rating Depression Scale (Zung 1965), Beck's Depression Inventory (Beck *et al* 1961) and the Hamilton Depression Scale (Hamilton 1960). These scales will be briefly described and discussed below.

The Zung Self Rating Depression Scale is a self-rating scale devised as an attempt to quantify the symptoms of depression, using the diagnostic criteria of the presence of a pervasive depressed affect, and its physiological and psychological concomitants as test items. The test consists of 20 items reflecting the characteristics of depression as detailed earlier. The items were selected from illustrative verbatim records from patient interview material. The scale is devised so that of the 20 items used, 10 are worded symptomatically positive, and ten symptomatically negative. Mean indices achieved on the scale for patients diagnosed as depressive disorders were 0.74. The mean index for patients who were initially diagnosed as depressive disorder, but discharged as suffering from some other disorder, was 0.53. The mean index for the

Assessment

non-depressed control group was 0.33. Few aphasic individuals would have sufficiently intact language skills to complete the Zung without considerable input from the examiner.

The Beck Depression Inventory, like the Zung, is a self-rating scale covering 21 areas of behaviour associated with depression. The subject is asked to read the statements covering each area and mark the most correct statement according to his or her feelings. Each statement has a point and the result is summarized. The sum indicates the degree of depression. Like the Zung, the Beck requires intact linguistic skills for successful completion.

The *Hamilton Depression Scale* is the most frequently used tool to quantify depressive symptoms. Unlike the Zung and the Beck, the technique used is an interview-based clinical rating completed by the examiner. It consists of 18 items and in some versions with operationalized scaled steps. The items cover the usual areas like insomnia, guilt feelings, mood, retardation, agitation, anxiety etc. Since this scale is in frequent use there are many different versions. The inter-rater reliability is, in most versions, good. In a Swedish version (Rubenowitz 1977) the inter-rater coefficient ratio varied between 0.75 - 0.91. While aphasic subjects may have difficulties in responding to the questions, the examiner can adjust and vary the language to elicit as full a response as possible.

The CPRS, discussed below, has a subscale for rating of depressive mood. This subscale consists of ten items which are very practical to use in clinical as well as in scientific work. The Visual Analogue Scale, discussed above, has been used to rate the degree of depression and mood in subjects (Folstein 1975).

A last word on depression scales. Interview-based rating scales have the advantage of being sensitive when utilized by trained examiners. Their effectiveness is limited with aphasic patients since all the instruments described above were originally designed for non-brain damaged persons with functional depressions. The variability in interview technique between examiners plays an important role and the difficulty of extrapolating a person's mood state in everyday life from a single interview is another limitation. The Hamilton Scale's validity is uncertain. In comparison with global ratings done by psychiatrists the results have been somewhat discouraging (Knesevich 1977). More encouraging is the fact that the VAS, the Zung and the Hamilton have been evaluated, in terms of validity and reliability, on brain damaged subjects. These scales have all been found to be both reliable and valid measures of depression in brain damaged subjects as determined by high correlation coefficients for inter-rater agreement, test-retest, and interscale correlation (Robinson and Benson 1981; Robinson and Szetala 1981; Robinson and Price 1982; Robinson *et al* 1983). The Beck involves the most difficult questions to read and is therefore not an appropriate instrument to use with dyslexic patients. The Zung scale is easier to read but in most studies the items have been read to the subjects. A more detailed critical review of depression scales is given in Carroll *et al* (1973).

The Comprehensive Psychopathological Rating Scale (CPRS).

This test was developed in Scandinavia by a group of psychiatrists, psychologists and clinical pharmacologists (Asberg *et al* 1978). The scale covers a broad range of psychopathological variables and can be used either in full or as a pool of items from which subscales can be drawn for particular psychiatric conditions. One of the subscales often used in clinical work and research with aphasic subjects is the depression scale. The scales consists of different sets of items (the depression scale consists of ten items), and the scale steps have been operationally defined. General rules have been applied in the construction of the scale in order to reach consistency. The examiner rates the patient during an interview and explicit instructions on how to obtain the necessary information from the subject are given in the text to each scale step. Two extra items are added in the end of the scale, one concerning the global rating of illness and the other concerning the reliability of the rating. The inter-rater reliability is reported high (Montgomery *et al* 1978), and the validity in comparison with a well-known and well-established Swedish depression scale, the Cronholm-Ottosson Depression Rating Scale (Cronholm and Ottosson, 1960), is reported as good.

Questionnaires

If we want to know how people feel: what they experience and what
they remember, what their emotions and motives are like, and the
reasons for acting as they do - why not ask them?
G.W. Allport (1942).

The questionnaire is likely to be a less expensive procedure in terms of skill and time than the interview. It requires much less skill to administer and they are often handed out to subjects with a minimum of explanation. Questionnaires can also be administered to large numbers of individuals simultaneously and they can be sent by mail. However, and most relevant for the purposes of this book, because most aphasics cannot usually understand the questions, the use of questionnaires is limited to gaining information from relatives. Even this information tends to be more complete if obtained during an interview but in the context of research the questionnaire has the advantage of being more standardized and reliable. In some cases the standardized questionnaire can be read to the aphasic subject and thereby fulfil the criterion on standardization. If there is little need for standardization, like in everyday clinical work, the interview will have the potential of providing much more information.

The term *questionnaire* is used for many different approaches. Sometimes the term is used to describe constructions of well established measurement techniques like the Thurstone scale, the Likert scale or the Guttman scale. These are all well defined procedures for the production of an attitude scale. In other cases the term questionnaire means a standardized questioning technique with fixed or open response alternatives. Sometimes the term indicates nothing more and nothing less than a sheet of paper with questions the examiner finds interesting to get answers on. An advantage of all kinds of well designed questionnaires is that the method is very direct; that is, one gets answers on the questions asked. This is also a limitation in the method since the subject is sometimes not aware of the attitudes or emotions the examiner is looking for. One way to get around this problem is to ask someone else who knows the subject well, like the spouse or a relative. There are other difficulties associated with questionnaires like, how much of the subject's response is influenced by his or her own attitudes and how much is repressed. The strategy of asking spouses to act as informants has been widely used in aphasia research for obvious reasons. The technique is valuable but great care should be exercised in the interpretation of data on one individual obtained from another. In some cases the data might be more informative about the spouse than the partner they were supposed to describe, but this information too can be valuable. For reasons discussed above it is important to account for how data has been collected.

The Code-Müller Protocols (CMP).

As we have discussed earlier in this book, it is probable that interpersonal factors can affect the rehabilitation outcome of the aphasic patient. In order to study these factors and elicit perceptions on psychosocial adjustment from patients, spouses and professionals, a set of 10 questions requiring a choice of rating by the subject was designed by Müller and Code (1983). This has come to be known as the *Code-Müller Protocols* (Code and Müller In Preparation). Questions are included on the ability to return to work, coping with depression, speaking to strangers, making new personal relationships and six others. The 10 questions are not intended to provide a comprehensive assessment of psychosocial perception are designed to sample perceptions. The protocols measure the extent to which there is agreement between one or more parties concerning future predictions about the degree of adjustment. In one study (Müller, Code and Mugford 1983), the authors found an incongruity of perceptions between therapists and spouses. The spouses appeared to be more optimistic about recovery.

The CMP constitute a useful clinical tool which can help guide counselling and rehabilitation. Little is known still about the ways in which different perceptions of the same problem might influence the rehabilitation outcome. The CMP are also valuable in highlighting different perceptions among aphasic patients, their spouses and the therapists.

The Personal Relations Index (PRI).
The PRI was developed by Mulhall (1977, 1978) as a psychological instrument for the exploration of some of the problems evolving from the interpersonal judgements of aphasic patients and their spouses. The instrument aims to construct a dynamic representation of the relationship between patient and spouse. The information is obtained through a clinical interview and if the patient cannot give the information, the spouse is used as informant. A graphical representation of a two-person relationship is produced as seen by one member of the interaction. The technique is not simple to grasp since several stages are involved, but potentially rich qualitative insights can be obtained of the dynamic interactions which take place between the parties. The following stages are described by Mulhall (1977):

1. During a free discussion the subject is asked to describe him or herself and the other person in the context of their relationship. These descriptions include attitudes, feelings or behavioural states which are referred to as elements.

2. The elements are fed into a computer program which produces a questionnaire unique to the subject. In answering the questionnaire the subject imposes order on his or her impressions by indicating how they are most likely to react to each of the other person's elements.

3. A graphical representation showing the dynamic interaction between the elements, and therefore the two people, is constructed by interconnecting each element with its most likely outcome(s).

4. This graphical representation is presented to the patient and spouse in a readily comprehensible form and enables them to understand better their own problem situation and hence aids them in resolving it.

5. Successive graphical representations of later states of affairs are also fed back to the subjects so that the improvements (in what is a complex dynamic situation) are apparent to them.

Mulhall (1978) found, using the PRI, that spouse's attempts to help and encourage the patient often increased the latter's frustration level. This attitude often resulted in the spouse, in turn, often responding negatively engendering another negative response from the patient and thereby creating a vicious circle.

The PRI has a dynamic quality that few other assessment scales can offer, but it is a rather difficult technique to use clinically. At the present time, where many clinicians are already overburdened with work, it might be to time-consuming to apply the technique in the clinical setting. Maybe this technique will be used more widely in clinical research in the future.

Assessment

Family diagnosis

As emphasized already, aphasia is not only an individual handicap but also has effects upon those who are near and dear the aphasic person. In particular, families are burdened by the sudden change in family life. Before going into discussion of procedures for investigation of the dynamics of the aphasic family, a framework will be outlined which will help provide us with a basis for understanding these complex processes.

A Basic Framework for Understanding Family Dynamics

The human family is a unique organization upon which modern society is built. Evidently the human being is a true familial animal. The family is devoted to protecting the biological integrity of the organism, but beyond this primary task the family has a main ongoing responsibility for the socialization of its members. The development of relationships (as discussed in Chapter 4) takes primarily place within the family, the mother and the father are in the beginning the representatives of the whole grown up world. The emotional significance of this experience will last for the rest of the young person's life.

Families are more than the sum of their members; families are held together by relationships which adds a further complex interactional dimension to the individual elements of the family. Families could be defined as a system depending on their members. The system is characterized by the elements (the family members), their attributes (qualities, personality traits, etc.) and the relationships which hold the system together.

Interaction between the family members - the elements - takes place through communication. All family systems have a direction; this direction might be functional or dysfunctional in relation to the purposes of each member. The direction of the

67

family system could be called *the family process*. The process is not always conscious to its members since it is a function of the family system rather than the individual members. Individual members of families can therefore sometimes find themselves caught up in an extremely destructive process, a process they have little understanding of since they sometimes have no awareness of the principles upon which the family process is working.

The features of family dynamics described above - the system's interactions, the role of communication, the family process, are fundamental to a useful understanding of family life (Lundsbye *et al* 1982). A sudden onset of illness, a disruption in communication or any other event that significantly interferes with the homeostasis of the family system, will be reflected in all areas of family life.

Family Assessment

To explore family functioning ideally requires methods which are rigorous in their design and application. As indicated in the previous section, families are extremely complex phenomena and methods are just beginning to be explored (Haley 1962). A good attempt to examine the different approaches and to develop the concept of family diagnosis was made by Hansson (1989). He describes four different theoretical approaches from the literature: an individual perspective based on a diagnosis which applies to one member (for instance aphasia), a generalized individual diagnosis (*the aphasic family*), a description of the system through one dimension (*expressed emotion, affective style* or *communication deviance*) and a description through several dimensions (*circumplex models*). Whatever theoretical approach is taken, a family interview or completion of specific tasks are used to collect information.

The family assessment or diagnosis should be based on a theoretical model that ultimately has an interventional perspective. Since work with families and the interactions of their members is based on different theoretical concepts it is impossible to reach a consensus in terms of diagnosis. Additionally, the examiner of *aphasic families* is restricted to the procedure normally utilized in family therapy.

Attempts have been made to assess marital satisfaction in families with an aphasic member. *The Marital Satisfaction Scale* (see Chapter 3) is one scale used for this purpose. It examines areas such as the respondent's satisfaction with the emotional support provided by the spouse, general lifestyles, and sexual relationships. The scale was first introduced by Roach *et al* (1981). A limitation of considerable importance is that the scale represents a statistical description of the relationship as seen by the spouse.

Another important feature of family assessment is described by Rollin (1984, 1987). He underlines the importance of evaluation of the aphasic individual's degree and quality of communicative impairment. This knowledge will assist the family therapist to acquire a more realistic view of the communication patterns existing in the family. Therapeutic intervention with families will be discussed in Chapter 6.

Management and Treatment of Psychological and Social Problems in Aphasics and Their Families

Approaches to Intervention

While methods of treatment abound for aphasia, there has been little work developing approaches for psychic and psychosocial problems, despite the fact that many speech pathologists have stressed the importance of giving the family members of aphasic patients the opportunity to participate in the rehabilitation process. While it should not be surprising to find emotional and social reactions in survivors, more surprising is the lack of attempts at intervention. In this chapter we will examine approaches to intervention with aphasic individuals and their families.

Fundamental Prerequisites for Rehabilitation

Rehabilitation after brain damage is a challenging assignment for patients, relatives and professionals. Comprehensive rehabilitation programmes must take into account both medical, social and psychological aspects. The World Health Organization (1980) has suggested in the International Classification of Impairment, Disability and Handicap a distinction between these different states:

impairment is described as a disturbance at the organic level;

> **disability** is measured by functional performance and activity restriction;

> **handicap** is measured in terms of the disadvantage in fulfilment of various roles in society.

Brain damage can result in impairments, disabilities and handicaps. For many aphasic patients all three apply.

Whatever terminology is used it should be remembered that the presenting somatic or psychic state can be interpreted from many different perspectives. Even though the physician might consider the patient as not severely handicapped, maybe because they are focused on comparing handicap between patients, the family or the patient can experience the situation completely differently. An early step in the rehabilitation process therefore, must be to clarify different perspectives on the situation, among doctors, speech pathologists, other carers, the family members and the patient. This raises an important question on the problem of determining degree of recovery. Should we measure recovery in terms of reduction in impairments, disabilities or handicaps? One approach must certainly be that the best rehabilitation results are those based on the point of view of the patient. If the patient experiences even a slight anomic aphasia as a severe handicap he or she will act in relationships and in the community as if they were severely handicapped. As detailed earlier, the opinion of family members on the handicap can influence rehabilitation outcome (see Chapter 3). An early and important phase in the rehabilitation process, therefore, will be to evaluate the patients difficulties from different perspectives.

A common requirement of a rehabilitation programme is to set **therapeutic goals** and the goals vary considerably from one patient to another. In many centres these goals are arrived at in meetings between professionals, significant others in the patient's social network, family members and the patient him/herself. Such meetings have the advantage of being a forum for discussion of different perspectives. While different perspectives are natural and unavoidable, it is of course very counterproductive if different involved individuals have different goals and different ambitions.

Planning for the longterm care of the brain damaged and the aphasic person must take into account some essential elements leading to some basic questions that must be answered:

1. Does the patient fully understand what has happened to him or her?

2. Has the patient a good home in the future which is adjusted to their needs?

3. Has the patient anything meaningful to do in the future?

4. Is there anyone who cares for the patient?

When the therapeutic programme is planned and the questions above are considered, the next phase will be to **realize the programme**. This should be done as soon as possible since prolonged immobilization and mental passiveness probably serve to only generate more disability.

Psychosocial Aspects of Recovery from Brain Damage

While a range of factors have been identified which are related to recovery of behavioural and cognitive functions, it is far from clear how these factors may inter-relate to influence recovery. We briefly examine physiological and psychosocial factors important in recovery in this section.

Physiological mechanisms underlying recovery from brain damage will be only superficially discussed here (for more detailed discussion see Laurence and Stein

1978 and Albert 1988). However, before going in to more detail on treatment of psychic and social problems in aphasics and their relatives, it is necessary to touch on the subject, since emotional and behavioural aspects of recovery are closely tied to physical recovery.

According to Woolsey (1978) a range of relevant changes can arise from a lesion: those caused by the lesion trauma itself; whether it's focal or diffuse; the kinds of neural degeneration involved; degeneration of neurochemical pools; the degree of vascular disruption; oedema and raised pressure in the cerebrospinal fluid.

Diaschisis may play an important role. This describes the process where the threshold of cells not directly affected by the lesion and at some distance from the lesion, rises considerably so that they cease to respond to normal strength stimulation and cease to function normally. Recovery from diaschisis is unpredictable in terms of time span (Luria 1963) and the relationship to emotional and behavioural changes in the patient is unclear but unspecific influences on psychic processes of recovery may take place.

Activation of relatively ineffective synapses is a fairly new concept in neurobiology. The concept suggests that activation of pre-existing connections that were dormant or originally ineffective partly accounts for what is generally called neural plasticity (Laurence and Stein 1978). Hypothetically this reorganisation might influence emotional and behavioural recovery in the sense that new strategies of coping are developed and a possible reorganisation of mood maintenance takes place.

Denervation supersensitivity describes the condition where a central neuron loses its afferents and thereby acquire *supersensitivity* to any residual transmitter that impinges upon it. Supersensitivity for dopaminergic and cholinergic systems arise at about one month after brain damage (Albert 1988). Noradrenergic and serotonergic systems are maximally supersensitive at six months to two years, paralleling the time course for depression (Robinson *et al* 1984). Albert (1988) has concluded from this that:

psychological, environmental or pharmacological measures which could
inhibit or reverse the tendency towards perseveration, depression or
epilepsy, especially if introduced at the appropriate time in the process
of recovery, should improve chances for effective aphasia rehabilitation
(p. 216).

We return to the role of pharmacological treatment at the end of this chapter.

As we have seen, recovery and adjustment following brain damage with aphasia is, to an extensive degree dependent on circumstances almost impossible to measure objectively. Environmental influences on recovery are considered important by most aphasic patients, according to the studies we have discussed, as well as social factors. But it is difficult to identify the beneficial aspects in a conventional scientific manner. However, some factors seem to be crucial in successful readjustment, like the provision of basic and correct information to patients and their relatives, good co-operation between the hospital and the family, a caring social network, and so on. Some of these factors will be discussed next.

A Residential Programme for Aphasic Families

Our group in Gothenburg has completed a series of studies which were designed to examine and evaluate psychotherapeutic intervention in the lives of patients and their spouses. Borenstein *et al* (1987a) arranged a five-day residential course outside the hospital for aphasic patients and their family members. The course was led by a speech pathologist, a psychologist and a neurologist. The aim of the course was to give the aphasics and their relatives information on etiology, treatment possibilities and prognosis of aphasia. The participating families underwent family therapy every day. Individual counselling with the aphasic as well as with the spouse was offered regularly during the course. In addition talks on different topics, such as local cultural history, geography, etc., were provided. The participants also met daily in different speech therapy groups led by the speech pathologist. Excursions and relaxation-exercises were also on the schedule. Patients were not grouped together with the members of their family in order to avoid overprotection. Each aphasic participant underwent linguistic, psychological and neurological examination. The course participants met again one year after the course for evaluation.

The study was carried out as a single group outcome study and data were reported in terms of intra-individual changes. Changes were noted in several areas like, knowledge about aphasia and the physical impairment, beliefs and attitudes toward the linguistic and physical impairment. A marked improvement in mood was found, both in the aphasics as well as in their family members. In summary a general improvement was noted and the authors concluded:

> *Through this process the families were given opportunities to verbalize experiences, feelings and thoughts to each other, including "hard" or "forbidden" feelings. The psychologist provided a permissive atmosphere, gave the family support, and also helped the family members to respond and take initiatives. This was done by letting them become sensitive to the non-verbal signs of the aphasic member and also by letting the sessions take time and allowing all possible forms of communication. From a therapeutic point of view, the benefits to family members included freedom to share their frustrations with each other, and the opportunity to react freely in a supportive atmosphere. Through this therapeutic process the family were able to deal more effectively with the new situation* (Borenstein *et al* 1987a: p. 55).

Since most of the participants in this course thought that the information given was positive and useful, it might be concluded that there should be fewer misconceptions within the families concerning the nature of aphasia and the repercussions upon individuals with aphasia and their relatives. Our presuppositions in this study about the context most suitable for assimilating the information seemed to be correct since the atmosphere was very relaxed and undramatic. The ongoing dialogue during the course between the hospital staff and the families gave opportunities to work through difficulties that are usually left for families to solve on their own, often with undesirable results. Our experience suggests that the method described seems to increase the potential of the aphasic person and the family to enjoy a more positive and effective rehabilitation and a better adjustment to disabilities.

This study can be criticised on the basis that the same changes may have occurred as a result of attention or other uncontrolled factors, since no control group was involved. This is always a problem with single group outcome studies, but at the time it was considered more important to make an attempt to investigate changes following the programme and it was not considered ethical to exclude some patients and their relatives from the information given, from family therapy or the individual counselling. In practice it is extremely difficult to develop a really meaningful control design for a study like this one.

Information to The Patient and The Family

We have noted in several places in this book that many aphasic individuals and their family members are not sufficiently informed about the impairment, its consequences and prognosis. This insufficiency has the potential to be counterproductive in the readjustment process. It is not sufficient to provide information once, either verbally or in the form of a leaflet. Information has to be given several times since most patients as well as their relatives are in a state of shock early post-onset. An effective programme for imparting information should be repeated at least once; once following onset and again a couple of months later. In order to ensure full understanding, the information should be repeated a third time, and this might be done as part of general information giving during the rehabilitation programme. It is even more beneficial for the individual aphasic and his or her family if they have a particular physician, speech pathologist or psychologist to turn to in cases of uncertainty. Such key positions of trust could be connected with the stroke club or aphasic patient association.

One way to ensure that useful and clear information for patients and families is reaching people, is to arrange courses like those described earlier. A couple of months after onset, when the giving of initial information will have been given, the patients and their families can be invited for a programme of three or four sessions where they are informed about medical, communicative, psychosocial and other important implications of the impairment. **It is not sufficient to just hand out a pamphlet to the relatives.** Often such pamphlets give rise to more questions than they answer. Pamphlets should be seen as complements to the main effort, but should not replace the careful provision of information given face to face with opportunities to ask more personal questions.

Co-operation

Co-operation is of central importance in rehabilitation. There are so many new things in life for the brain damaged and their relatives to adjust to that co-operation is absolutely essential between all those involved in the rehabilitation process, in order to make the adjustment easier for the patient. A co-operative team approach from the professionals involved and a planned rehabilitation programme involving the patient and their relatives, makes it possible to avoid unnecessary hardship for patient and relatives. After the patient has left the hospital it is important for them to keep contact with the professional team. Physiotherapists, occupational therapists, speech pathologists, and so on, need to share their experiences and knowledge about the patient even when the patient has become an outpatient. Furthermore, it is important to establish a working relationship between the patient, the family and a social worker who can take care of and guide the family in practical aspects of coping.

Patient Associations

Some Western countries have Patient Associations of some kind. From experience these organisations have meant a lot to the patients as well as their families. According to Linell and Steg (1980, p. 89) such an organisation should have certain objectives. They suggested the following:

> To increase knowledge of the syndromes of aphasia amongst patients and relatives as well as in society as a whole.

> To work for increased contact between members of the association through meetings, excursions, clubs, and study groups, etc.

> To support research in the field.

> To work for better resources in society and within the hospital system for the rehabilitation of patients with aphasia.

Support and Psychotherapy

The type of psychotherapy provided to an individual is dependent on the theoretical beliefs held by the practitioner. Different schools have been developed from the Freudian tradition, the behaviourist tradition, the existentialist tradition, the interactionist tradition, and so on. Within these theoretical frameworks different practical techniques have been developed. Even the time course of therapy varies according to different theories and strategies adopted by the therapist. It is important to distinguish support programmes from psychotherapy since the latter method has the major aim of *changing* internal psychic structures while the former aims at *supporting* the individual's own strengths through counselling. Practising psychotherapy requires professional knowledge and skills and should not be undertaken without proper training. Support is, of course, something everyone can give and practice. (See Brumfitt and Clarke 1989 for discussion of psychotherapy with aphasic individuals.)

Support Programmes

A variety of support programmes have been described earlier in this book (see Chapters 2, 5 and 6). The research discussed suggests that support programmes can be important and effective elements in a comprehensive rehabilitation process. Support programmes can be offered to the patients, the relatives and both. The composition of the group should be dictated by the aims of the group. It is therefore important to make the aims explicit before starting a group.

Rice *et al* 1987) reported a marked improvement in spouses with aphasic partners after participation in a social support group. The aim of the group was to offer emotional support and relevant information. They undertook a comparison between good and poor attenders. *Good* attenders were those who were able to attend the group regularly (an average of 10 out of 12 occasions), the *poor* attenders were those who, due to personal circumstances, attended less regularly (an average of 2 out of 12 occasions). Good attenders showed significant improvement at various stages on tests of social dysfunction, somatic symptoms, anxiety, and in a broad measure of psychological well-being (the PRI discussed in Chapter 5). Some functional improvement in the partners of good attenders was also noted. The authors concluded that participation in a support group is of psychological benefit to spouses of aphasic patients.

Certain elements seem to be important in support groups. It is an advantage if the support group can **meet regularly** since the group for a period of time can offer an **experiential opportunity** and **participatory involvement** to the participants. In other words, a given place and time for the psychological and social encounter with a new situation in life. The support group can give both the aphasic person and/or the relatives the opportunity to **develop and improve interpersonal communication and relationships** through a natural experiential process. Another element, already discussed, is the opportunity in such a group to **give and share information**. In such a permissive group atmosphere, not only the formal *facts* are discussed by an expert, but also the informal and natural exchange of personal experience can take place amongst the members. Activities can include role play games or other social activities that can help encourage personal growth. Informal social activities can be used, like listening to music, painting, discussion of a topic, or other activities chosen to encourage personal growth, inter-personal communication and self-awareness.

Family Therapy

Using the techniques of family therapy with aphasic families is a new approach to intervention for emotional and psychosocial problems following aphasia (Rollin 1987, 1988; Währborg 1989; Währborg and Borenstein 1990). Family therapy should be regarded as an outgrowth of psychotherapy and is thereby distinguished from family support groups or other forms of supportive intervention in family life. The aims of family therapy in families with an aphasic member can be summarized as follows:

1. To explore cognitive and emotional patterns of the family before, during and after onset of aphasia in a family member.

2. To teach the family about the handicap and common reactions

associated with it.

3. To encourage and reinforce emotional sharing in the family and guide its members in the process of acting out grief, anger, frustration, etc.

4. To bring up common issues faced in these families and introduce open and direct communication on delicate topics such as sexuality, bodily changes, etc.

5. To encourage the aphasic family member to explain what kind of help he or she wants from the other members of the family, such as if and when they want help with verbal cueing.

6. To teach the family how to time their interactions differently.

7. To teach family members to notice nonverbal communication behaviour, especially emotional qualities and to check and clarify their interpretations.

8. To teach special feedback techniques if the aphasic family member suffers from apraxia, impaired control of affect or impaired motivation.

9. To recommend to the family to refrain from formal linguistic training of their partner unless they have been specifically asked to by the speech pathologist.

The techniques used in family therapy are based on systems theory, communication theory and process theory. However, some features of family therapy with aphasic families are very special and need to be discussed here. We examine these special features below while looking at an outline of the basic structure of a family therapy programme.

Since one of the members of the therapy group is aphasic the therapy has to be structured and strategic; i.e. the therapist has to initiate what happens during the therapy and design the particular approach to each problem. It is important to note at the start that the focus should be on *the family* and not the aphasic family member.

The social phase. Here the therapist and the family members get to know each other and the therapist is developing relationships and laying the foundations for a therapeutic atmosphere. This is achieved by emphasizing positive aspects of the family based on the assumption that there is a desire for growth within all persons.

The explorative phase. Here the therapist explores the communicative possibilities and potential within the family. The therapist finds out in what way he or she can communicate with the aphasic member but also with the other family members. It is important that everybody in the family discover different ways of communication. The focus should not be on the aphasic person only.

The problem-orienting phase. This is where the therapist interviews each family member in order to find out what they are dissatisfied with, what they want to change, how they want to do it and when. During this part of the interview the therapist is practising a variety of therapeutic techniques to make communication open and clear. One technique is *clarification*; i.e. using questions aimed at making a statement comprehensible and understandable, identifying the feelings and intentions involved. The therapists approach obviously depends on the communication capabilities of the respondent. The technique is also a way of checking out a message with the sender (see example below).

The diagnostic phase. By now the therapist has been able to recognize aspects of the family system (who starts to answer open questions, who acts as the head of the family, who is dominant, who is subservient, etc.). The therapist can now also note individual styles and patterns in communication or incongruence in the communication process. The dysfunctional processes in the family, causing psychic and psychosocial disorder, start to become clearer for the trained therapist.

The therapeutic phase. In this final phase, the therapist picks out one problem or process in the family and starts to work with it. A variety of verbal and nonverbal therapeutic techniques are available at this point, encounter techniques and others.

To illustrate the principles of family therapy outlined above we will examine an example of a sequence in a family therapy session with a rather young couple. The wife has had a subarrachnoidal haemorrhage and she has acquired a right sided hemi-paresis and Broca's aphasia. The severity of the aphasia is moderate. The wife has attempted suicide and they both agreed to participate in family therapy. We can call them Liz and Tom. The dialogue is picked up in the *therapeutic* phase of the therapy.

Therapist (T): Tom, you said that you care for your wife. Does that mean that she can do what she wants?

Tom: I mean, I care for her..... I still love her .... I don't want her to drink that much. Who knows, maybe that is one of the reasons she got that haemorrhage.

T: You didn't answer my question.

Tom: What question?

T: If she can do what she wants.

(Liz follows the conversation intensely with her eyes.)

Tom: Of course not. I think she is drinking to much.

(Liz turns her head away. There is a smile on her lips.)

T: Tom look at your wife now....... What can you see?

Tom: She is not interested.

T: Interested in what?

Tom: Interested in what we are talking about.

T: (touching Liz) Liz, are you interested in this matter?

(Liz is nodding)

T: (looking at Tom) She is interested.

Tom: It doesn't look like she is.

T: Tom what do you think your wife is feeling right now?

Tom: (looking at his wife, then at the therapist, he pauses...) I don't know.

T: Ask her.

Tom: (looking in the roof)

T: You won't get any answers from there.

Tom: No, I know .... Say it Liz, what do you feel?

(Liz is lifting her left arm and with her hand she is making a gesture to cut her throat).

T: Tell me Tom, what do you feel now?

(Tom get tears in his eyes and turns his head away from the therapist and Liz. The therapist stands up and gently turns Liz's head towards Tom).

T: Tom, tell Liz what you feel.

Tom: (with tears in his eyes and broken voice) I love you Liz.... You make me so scared......I don't want to lose you.

(Liz looks down at the floor)

T: (turning to Liz) Did you here Tom?

Liz: Yes.

T: Did you like what he said, that he loved you?

Liz: (looking at Tom) ......Yes ....I ...did.

T: (turning to Liz) Is it important for you to be able to do what you want to do?

(Liz is nodding)

T: Even to take a drink when you want?

(Liz is nodding again)

T: (turning to Tom) Could you see and hear that Tom. Liz thinks that it is important for her to able to do what she want to do.

This dialogue is an example of a therapeutic process between two individuals, one of whom is aphasic. The aphasia requires certain knowledge and training on the part of the therapist to handle but otherwise there is no difference between family therapy with an aphasic family and in other families with problems.

Währborg and Borenstein (1989) examined the usefulness of family therapy in families with an aphasic member. In this study 37 family members and 22 aphasic patients participated. They were studied before and six months after the therapy with standardized interviews. During the interview the subject was asked to grade the changes that had taken place in the other person (aphasic or family member) since onset on a five-point scale. The interview questionnaires (one for the family members and one for the aphasic subjects) consisted of 22 and 18 items, and covered fives areas: emotions, behaviour, social life, communication and medical problems.

The result suggested that family therapy has a beneficial impact on aphasic family life. Most changes occurred in the aphasic patients themselves. After family therapy, depression, emotional isolation, impatience and social isolation diminished in the patients and knowledge about the handicap increased in both patients and in their relatives.

The authors concluded that:

family therapy has the potential to develop new and important communication skills in aphasic families. The decrease in tendency toward depression, especially in the aphasics is related to the use of structured techniques to develop psychologically important communication skills. The aphasic person needs to be the recipient of emotional responses and reactions she or he cannot ask for. Family therapy is a psychological technique that can meet this need. Family therapy also provides the family and the aphasic with a natural opportunity to share and act out emotions. In this study only between two and six sessions of family therapy were offered. It is possible that an increased number of sessions and a prolongation of them might further improve the outcome. Despite the limited number of sessions it is particularly noteworthy that patients perceive that their relatives learn more about the handicap. The results of this study suggest that family therapy is a beneficial part of the rehabilitation process for aphasics and their families (Währborg and Borenstein 1989).

The aphasic state cannot be changed by family therapy but the quality of communication can. For more detailed discussion of the procedures of family therapy and for an overview of the basic principles see Walrond-Skinner (1976) and for application with aphasic families see Rollins (1987, 1988) and Währborg (1989) and accompanying commentaries to Währborg.

Group Therapy

Group therapy is usually based on the same principles as family therapy, but the group dynamics are different. Most studies on group work (see Chapter 2) with aphasic individuals have employed group counselling programmes. These programmes are more support groups than psychotherapy groups.

In 1950 Nathan Blackman published an anecdotal paper on group psychotherapy with aphasic patients. He claimed that the programme was beneficial and reported positive changes in each case. Turnblom and Myers (1952) described a group discussion programme for the families of aphasic individuals. Based on the written and verbal comments of the participants, the authors suggest that a group counselling programme helped the families to adjust emotionally to the problems arising. Derman and Manaster (1967) describe a four-session family counselling programme based on short lectures about physical and psychological problems connected with aphasia. They also distributed a publication, *Aphasia and the Family*, to the families they worked with. The first session offered information and the other three were more *therapeutic*. The group evolved into an open-ended continuing group available to relatives of aphasic outpatients and inpatients. Anecdotally, the authors reported more realistic and accepting attitudes in the relatives as a result of the programme.

Emerson (1980) studied the changes in depressive states and self-esteem in spouses of stroke patients with aphasia through group counselling. A pre- and post-test control group design was used that allowed 11 spouses to volunteer for a treatment or control group. Six spouses (four female and two male) volunteered for the treatment group and five spouses (four female and one male) volunteered for the control group. The groups were similar in important demographic variables and in pretest results. Although significant changes were not found between the groups in the post-test scores, Emerson still concluded that an eclectic treatment programme that stresses the developmental and personal mastery approach to group work has a strong therapeutic potential.

Since the experiences of group psychotherapy with aphasic patients are limited one can only speculate on the advantages of the technique. Group psychotherapy has the potential to illuminate the human personality in a multidimensional way and provide for a deeper understanding of the aphasic person or his or her relatives through the quality of the aphasic person's relationships to the other group members and the therapist. For the aphasic person it provides representation of a microcosmos, or a segment of the real world, and as such it represents an important existential encounter for the participants. Group psychotherapy has the potential to liberate many aphasics from their *idios cosmos* - their tendency to get bound-up and lost in themselves. Many aphasic persons as well as others who have experienced a severe trauma become self-centred or egocentric, wasting a lot of energy on reliving the traumatic experience and the consequences of it. Confrontation with others in the same situation might enable the aphasic person to live in the *koinos cosmos* - the shared world of communing. Our understanding of the role of these complex dynamics and processes in aphasia will be improved by further studies on group psychotherapy with aphasic persons in the future.

Individual Psychotherapy

Psychotherapy is a generic term and it is inaccurate to talk of psychotherapy as a specific form of treatment. There are a variety of different techniques, some based on well defined presuppositions and theories and others on no theory at all. Individual psychotherapy with aphasics is no different than psychotherapy with other people in this sense. However, approaches to individual psychotherapy share some common features (Frank 1972, p. 38):

1. An intense, emotionally charged, confiding relationship with a helping person.

2. A rationale or myth which includes an explanation of the cause of the person's distress and a method for relieving it. To be effective, the therapeutic myth must be compatible with the cultural world-view shared by the patient and therapist. The supplying of a conceptual scheme, for what seems to the patient to be a group of nonsensical symptoms, provides powerful reassurance. It is the function of the rationale and technique rather than their specific content and form which really count.

3. Provision of new information concerning the nature and sources of the patient's problems and alternative ways of dealing with them.

4. Strengthening the patient's expectations of help through the personal qualities of the therapist, enhanced by his or her status in society and the setting in which he or she works.

5. Provision of the experience of successful mastery over symptoms which heighten the patient's hopes.

6. Facilitation of emotional arousal, a prerequisite of attitudinal and behavioural change.

All six features contribute to the effectiveness of individual psychotherapy. To treat aphasic people with psychotherapy requires special qualities from the therapist and care in the choice of techniques:

1. The therapist should be trained in aphasiology. Without knowledge or experience of aphasia, general consequences of brain damage and the patient's linguistic limitations, the therapist would not be able to make proper use of different communicative modalities available. The therapist might also misunderstand behavioural expressions in the patient.

2. The therapy technique used should be explained and understood by the aphasic patient who should accept the psychotherapeutic treatment by their own free will.

3. The aphasic patient should have an ability to appreciate that the

things that are going to be explored are psychological in nature and should express a willingness to explore him- or herself.

4. The techniques adopted must accommodate the uniqueness of the aphasic patient and therefore allow all kinds of communicative expressions.

The effectiveness of psychotherapy on emotional and behavioural symptoms in aphasics has not yet been proven, either as psychoanalytic, neo-Freudian, existential or behaviour therapy. An interesting application to aphasia is described by Brumfitt and Clarke (1989).

The Grief Reaction

As already discussed, going through a psychic or social trauma can produce a mixture of feelings; frustration, grief, hopelessness, etc. Becoming aphasic and sometimes hemiplegic is of course a severe trauma. Some reactions that appear may be due to the lesion *per se*, as discussed earlier, but to some extent the reaction to the trauma is a natural reaction. As we have seen, differentiating the etiologies is difficult even with professional training, but to understand the human reactions to a trauma of this magnitude takes no more than natural human common sense. A grief reaction can result from the sudden onset of a situation for which the individual has no coping strategies. The grief is therefore limited to **a traumatic experience**; i.e. an unexpected situation of great emotional significance and it should not be confused with the prolonged emotional reaction to a trauma. The prolonged reaction is dependent on a more complete set of psychological variables and differs markedly between people. The grief reaction appears to have a universal dimension. Different variants of the model have been described by a number of authors (Kubler-Ross 1969; Tanner and Gerstenberger 1989 and accompanying commentaries). The model presented here is partly adopted from Cullberg (1975). The grief reaction has been described in the following phases:

1: The shock state.

This initial phase is characterized by a state of shock: an almost paralysed state, where the patient does not seem to fully have understood what has happened. Typical of this phase is the obvious psychic unpreparedness characterized by latency in emotional reaction. A variety of defence mechanisms (repression, suppression, regression, denial, projection, isolation and rationalization) might sometimes act as protection against the painful realization of the trauma. In the shock state the person is unprepared and has no tried and tested patterns of coping response. If the individual remains locked in this phase, a state of hysteria can result. In the natural course of crises the state of shock diminishes and leaves room for the next phase.

2: The reactive phase.

In this phase the significance of the trauma suddenly becomes very apparent. This insight has two dimensions, a primary and a secondary. For example, a little boy falls off his bicycle onto the street. At first he does not seem to react at all (shock state), but after a while, maybe in his mothers arms, he starts to cry (*primary reaction*). Later, looking at his severely damaged cycle and suddenly discovering a new dimension to the trauma, he realizes that he cannot use it any more, and he cannot get it back. He develops a *secondary reaction* of depression. This depression is transient and a natural reaction to the loss. The aphasic person has lost something more important than the little boy's bicycle, but he or she reacts principally in the same way. The primary reaction is often frustration, especially in Broca's patients, but after some time the frustration is succeeded by a transient depression. A prolonged affective disorder can be a legacy of this phase (but can also be due to a direct result of the brain damage of course).

3. The reasonable phase.

This phase is characterized by the question why? Why did this happen? Why did it happen to me? Why did I not go to the doctor before? All these questions are usually parts of a beginning process of understanding and acceptance. Sometimes it might indicate the beginning of a chronic neurotic state with the development of all kinds of minor psychiatric symptoms. In the healthy, natural course of the grief response this phase constitutes a process of development and maturation, even though it is a painful experience.

4. The reorientation phase

This phase is characterized by orientation towards the future. The acute crisis is left behind and the emotional reaction has developed into a new preparedness. The crisis is no longer a crisis but an experience, integrated into the persons mental life.

The states described above should not be *treated* since they are not really an expression of disorder. From a professional point of view the grief reaction becomes a disorder when it departs from the natural course. In these cases the grief reaction is a part of the etiology and no longer a functional process in the mental maturation. One can guide and counsel a person through crises but this is not the same as to treat an emotional disorder. The guidance process should include support and help to identify the emotional content of the trauma; i.e. to support the person's own resources to cope. This support might also include mobilization of exterior resources such as the family, friends and other significant persons. Sometimes it is satisfactory just to be present, to listen and to allow time to take its course.

The natural course of a grief reaction described above is something most of us go through several times in life. The reactions are natural and healthy. This fact is worded by Lessing (in Schatzman 1974) in a memorable aphorism:

Wer Uber gewisse Dinge den Verstand nicht verliert, der hat keinen zu verlieren

(Those who do not lose their mind, sometimes have no mind to lose).

A Programme for Young Aphasic Adults

Younger aphasic individuals are given little particular attention in the research literature. Since the experiences from the programme described above were positive it was decided to initiate a more comprehensive study, based on the same basic principles, but addressing the particular problems of young aphasic people (Borenstein *et al* 1987b).

Eight relatively young aphasic adults (Median Age = 39.5 years) with a mean time post onset of three years were integrated into the normal curriculum at a Folk High School. These schools, which are unique to Scandinavia and Finland, determine their own course of study. The pupils live at the school and therefore spend a lot of time together. More emphasis is placed on developing co-operation, activity, independence and personality, than on formal schooling. The aphasic participants were assessed at the beginning, during and at the end of the course. Aphasia profiles were obtained through the Reinvang test (Reinvang and Engvik 1980), which is a standardized Swedish version of the Boston Diagnostic Aphasia Examination (Goodglass and Kaplan 1972). Verbal performance was examined using the Verbal Performance Rating Scale (Währborg and Borenstein 1988) which is a clinical rating scale for measuring functional language. Depression was measured with the Comprehensive Psychopathological Rating Scale (Asberg *et al* 1978), neuroticism with the Eysenck Personality Inventory (Eysenck and Eysenck 1964) and short-term memory using Luria's (1973) procedures. This study too was a single group outcome study since it was impossible to find any more young aphasic people in Sweden at the time who were willing to take part in any kind of control group.

The results of the study were very promising. It is worth noting that 7 out of 8 participants with aphasia for many years showed an improvement in their aphasia on Reinvang's test (see Figure 4). Verbal performance increased significantly from the first to the third test for most subjects. Improvement in mood was noticed but no changes were found in neuroticism, where the participants had an average of normal values from the beginning. The simple memory test showed no change (see Figure 5).

The uniqueness of this programme was that it let the aphasic students concentrate on an educational programme where they focused their mental and linguistic efforts on the acquisition of new knowledge rather than working on their individual aphasic symptoms.

Figure 4: Aphasic Profiles at the Start and Finish of the Course

Expressed as percentile points based on Reinvang's test (Reinvang and Engvik 1980).
Continuous lines = pre-test, dashed lines = post-test. F=fluency, A=auditory comprehension, R=repetition, N=naming, Q=aphasia quotient.

CASE 1: pre-test=transcortical motor aphasia, post-test=drop out

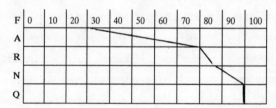

CASE 2: pre-test=discrete aphasic symptoms, post-test=discrete aphasic symptoms

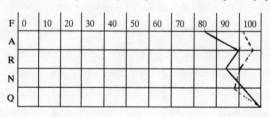

(Continued on next page)

CASE 3: pre-test=mixed fluency & impaired comprehension, post-test=conduction aphasia

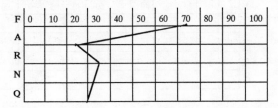

CASE 4: pre-test=nonfluent & severe comprehension impairment; post-test=improved comprehension

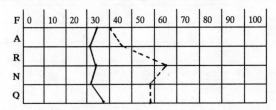

CASE 5: pre-test=nonfluent & impaired comprehension, post-test=conduction aphasia

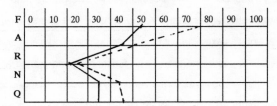

CASE 6: pre-test=transcortical motor aphasia, post-test=transcortical motor aphasia

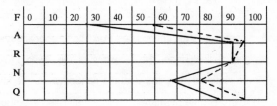

(Continued on next page)

CASE 7: pre-test=conduction aphasia, post-test=discrete aphasic symptoms

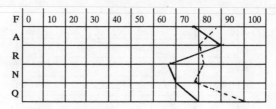

CASE 8: pre-test=mild Wernicke's aphasia, post-test=mild Wernicke's aphasia

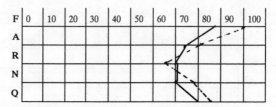

Since the young aphasics were integrated into the school with other young people without language difficulties, they were *forced* to use their own language to acquire new knowledge and also in daily life situations. The programme evidently had a significant therapeutic impact on the young aphasic participants.

Each participant was examined at the beginning, the middle and end of the course. In VPRS and CPRS score (indicating bad functional performance and pronounced depression) is 30. Improvement was recorded in both. Changes in the Eysenck Personality Inventory is presented in stan-nine-points. The inventory examines extroversion (E) and neuroticism (N) and has an in-built liescale (L) reflecting how much the testee tries to manipulate the answers. Memory results are given as median raw scores.

Since this study was published several new Folk High Schools have started similar courses for young aphasics' under the auspices of the Swedish Aphasia Patient Association. The educational programme at the school where the study took place is still active and now runs on a permanent basis; it has been extended and some of the aphasic young people have continued their education at the school.

Figure 5: Results of psychological examination at the beginning, middle and end of the course

Case	VPRS			CPRS			Eysenck									Memory		
							L	E	N	L	E	N	L	E	N			
1	11			13			3	5	6							5		
2	3.5	1.5	0	4.5	1.5	3	7	4	6	7	5	5	7	5	5	5	5	5
3	6	15.5	3.5	5.5	3.5	4	6	2	6	2	4	5	3	3	5	5	5	5
4	7.5	4	3	4	4.5	8	4	6	6	5	6	6	4	5	3	3	4	4
5	4	7.5	4	15	7	5	5	3	5	5	4	5	8	5	3	5	5	5
6	8.5	4	5	3.5	4	2	7	5	4	6	4	4	6	5	5	5	5	5
7	1	0.5	0.5	1.5	2.5	0	7	7	2	6	4	2	7	7	3	5	5	5
8	3	2.5	0.5	2	0.5	5	6	6	8	3	5	7	5	3	5	5	5	5
Md	4	4	4	3.5	4	3	7	5	5	6	4	5	7	5	3			
	$p=0.094$			$p=0.469$			No significant changes											
		$p=0.016*$			$p=0.125$													

Pharmacological Treatment

A general precaution obtains when prescribing drugs to brain damaged patients. Supersensitivity and other mechanisms might modify or mediate altered sensitivity to drugs. Only a few studies have been presented with impressive results on emotional and behavioural recovery following drug administration to aphasics. Nortriptyline has been shown to be efficient in treating post-stroke depression (Lipsey *et al* 1984). In a double-blind trial by Reding *et al* (1986) trazodone hydrochloride (Desyrel) with a target dose of 200 mg/daily was found to be associated with an improvement in Barthel activities of daily living scores. The authors concluded that patients with stroke and evidence of depression are likely to benefit from treatment with trazodone. A variety of drugs have been tried with aphasic individuals to improve language functions (Albert 1988). Former attempts include cashews and caffeine, without success. Modern attempts include dopamine, dopamine agonists and cholinergic drugs aimed at influencing neurotransmission. As yet these endeavours have produced little encouragement, but there are indications that this field may have a complementary role with other forms of therapy in the future.

Chapter 7

Long-term Evolution of Psychosocial and Emotional State.

Survivors of stroke and brain damage face a number of difficulties during the rehabilitation process. But most often it is believed that these problems decline with the passage of time. The natural history of recovery after brain damage has been presumed to proceed towards increased function and an improvement in most areas. Indeed this may be true to a some extent, but unfortunately this does not appear to be the case in recovery from the psychosocial and emotional consequences of brain damage. The indications are that these difficulties may not only persist for long after brain injury (Lundholm *et al* 1975; Najenson *et al* 1974; Thomsen 1984; Wåhrborg and Borenstein 1988b) but persisting deficits have been reported to be even worse after five years (Brooks *et al* 1986).

There appears to be a relationship between psychological deterioration and time in stroke patients. Wåhrborg and Borenstein (1988b) found a significant association between psychological deterioration and time for both aphasic and non-aphasic stroke patients (see Table 2).

The negative factors that turned out to be most correlated with time were dysphoric mood, tiredness, concentration capacity, anxiety and difficulties in taking initiatives. The aphasic subjects differed from the non-aphasics in some ways: they tended to more easily become irritated and touchy and tended to have a more reduced self-esteem.

In Table 2 an obvious difference can be seen between the variables so that some seem to be more responsible for the deterioration than others. Dysphoric mood and the tendency to become tired during the day were most related with time in this study. It should be noted that the questions were asked in Swedish and different keywords, more adapted to an every-day language, were used.

Table 2. Relationship between psychological deterioration and time in aphasic and non-aphasic stroke patients divided into separate variables and compared between the groups.

	Psychological deterioration vs. time		Difference between groups*
1. Are you often dysphoric?	$F=7.36$	$p<0.01$	NS
2. Do you find it hard to take initiative?	$F=2.69$	NS	NS
3. Do you easily get irritated?	$F=1.89$	NS	$p=0.99$
4. Do you easily become tired during the day?	$F=5.88$	$p<0.05$	NS
5. Do you find it hard to concentrate on things?	$F=3.97$	NS	NS
6. Do you easily become touchy?	$F=1.80$	NS	$p=0.99$
7. Do you at any time find you self-esteem degrading?	$F=0.20$	NS	$p=0.98$
8. Are you often worried?	$F=1.89$	NS	NS
9. Do you experience anxiety sometimes?	$F=3.10$	NS	NS
10. Do you easily forget?	$F=0$	NS	NS
11. Do you avoid social contact?	$F=0.30$	NS	NS

* Pitman's permutation test

The results led the authors to conclude that aphasic individuals, and stroke patients in general, are the victims of a spiralling process where an individual is deteriorating as a result of negative reinforcement and inadequate rehabilitation. Primary emotional and behavioural changes (caused directly by the brain damage) might be interpreted by relatives and care-givers as natural, secondary, psychological reactions and their

100

response to the individual is therefore based on a false belief. This fundamental misunderstanding about the nature of the handicap might result in demands and expectations of the aphasic person that he or she is not able to cope with. This process in combination with the effects of a communication breakdown in the family is the fuel in this dysfunctional process. The same deterioration is found in patients with traumatic etiology (Brooks *et al*. 1986). The aphasic person has not only the linguistic, the physical and the psychosocial problems to contend with, but also the combination of them; a combination that dominates all aspects of the individual's life and is most counterproductive in the struggle for recovery.

Why is this somewhat surprising and certainly discouraging psychological deterioration observed in aphasic and non-aphasic brain damaged patients? One possibility is that there are certain aspects of the patient's life that actually constitute a negative, counter-productive, dysfunctional *rehabilitation* process. As discussed earlier, when an individual suffers sudden damage to the brain there are effects on the person's emotional life. Of course the brain damage also causes immediate impairments of cognition and behaviour also which are not the primarily focus of this book. These impairments of language, perception and movement are *changes* which affect behaviour, but they also reduce the persons capacity to **express their personality**. There are good reasons to believe that the damage not only changes personality but the sudden onset of a communication impairment also restricts the individual's freedom to express him or herself. This means that, immediately following damage, the person undergoes changes as a result of primary and secondary factors.

An additional long-term influence comes from the family or other close relatives of the individual. The relatives are burdened by their reactions to the sudden changes in their own lives. They may go through some kind of a grieving process and then face a new set of circumstances that they are forced to live with and to deal with. This may be characterised by a prolonged period of sorrow where they miss the former person - the person who existed before the trauma, and the development of an unrealistically optimistic attitude. The sorrow and the missing process has at least two important components. Firstly the sorrow and the missing is directed towards the patient, the feelings are empathic. But after some time the feelings of sorrow and missing then also include grief for one's own lost person, i.e. the person they were before the traumatic changes occurred. During this prolonged period of sorrow and missing for the brain damaged person a new optimistic, and sometimes unrealistic, attitude takes form. This attitude might be seen as emotional *peptalk* rather than a realistic struggle for rehabilitation.

It appears therefore, that some years after onset the brain damaged individual enters a process of developing realization about the nature of their impairments. Sometimes, where patients are going through such a period of realization, but the family is still in a state of optimism about the future, there may be conflict. When family expectations are not congruent with what the patient experiences there can be a deterioration in the situation. The patient can react to such external conflicts with aggravation of the depressive mood or development of other psychological problems. During the realization period the patient is most vulnerable to attitudes in the family or in the environment. It is common for many brain damaged patients with major post stroke depression to develop a reactive depressive state as a result of this process.

In summary, we have suggested that a negative spiralling process develops in brain damaged persons which might be due to:

a) a lesion-induced psychiatric disorder or vulnerability;

b) a dysfunctional coping pattern in the patient and/or the family;

c) a natural response to the lesion-induced psychiatric disorder;

d) a natural reaction to unrealistic attitudes and dysfunctional coping patterns within the family;

e) a lack of support in psychological and social rehabilitation;

f) a concentration in rehabilitation programmes on overt elements of the handicap.

These factors, which may lead to long-term emotional or psychosocial problems for patient and family, need to be considered in rehabilitation management.

In this little book I have tried to bring together information on emotional and psychosocial reactions to aphasia for aphasic individuals, their relatives and others in their life. I have tried to provide guidance on the nature and cause of these problems and information on approaches to assessment and management. Good rehabilitation is hard work for patient, family and professionals. It is hard work for the patient to become a full member of society and leave an identity behind. This struggle deserves all our admiration since it is often a daily battle for what most of us take for granted - the right to be seen, and to be heard, and to make contact.

REFERENCES

Agren, H. 1980. Symptom patterns in unipolar and bipolar depression correlating with monoamine metabolites in the cerebrospinal fluid: 1. general patterns. *Psychiatric Research*, 3. 211-233.

Aitken, R.C.B. 1969. Measurement of feelings using visual analogue scales. *Proceedings and Research in Social Medicine* 69, 989-993

Albert, M. 1988. Neurobiological aspects of aphasia therapy. *Aphasiology* 2, 215-218.

Albert, M., Bachman, D., Morgan, A., and Helm Estabrook, N. 1987. Pharmacotherapy for aphasia. *Neurology* 37 (Supplement 1) 175.

Alford, L.B. 1933. Localization of Consciousness and Emotion. *American Journal of Psychiatry* 89, 789.

Allport, G.W. (1942) The use of personal documents in psychological science. *Bulletin 49, *Social Science Research Council*, USA.

Apt, P. and Kitzing, P. 1987. Incidens och omhändertagande av afasi i Sverige. Stencil. Talvärdsavdelningen, Malmö Allmänna Sjukhus.

Artes, R.H. 1967. A study of family problems as identified and evaluated by wives of stroke patients. *The University of Iowa. Department of Speech Pathology*.

Asberg, M., Montgomery, S., Perris, C., Schalling, D. and Sedvall, G. 1978. The Comprehensive Psychopathological Rating Scale. *Acta Psychiatrica Scandinavica*, Supplement 271.

Babinski, J. 1922. Reflexes de defense. *Brain* 45, 149-184.

Baldessarini, R.J. 1975. The basis for amine hypothesis in affective disorders. *Archives of General Psychiatry* 32, 1087-1093.

Bard, P. 1934. Emotion I. The neuro-humoral basis of emotional reactions. In: Murchinson, C. (Ed.,) *Handbook of General Experimental Psychology*. Worcester, Mass.: Clark University Press.

Bardach, J.C. 1969. Group sessions with wives of aphasic patients. *International Journal of Group Psychotherapy* 19, 361-365.

Bay, E. 1962. Aphasia and non-verbal disorders of language. *Brain* 85, 411-426.

Beck, A.T., Ward, C.H., Mendelson, M., Mock, J. and Erbaugh, J. 1961. Inventory for measuring depression. *Archives of General Psychiatry* 4, 53-63.

Benson, D.F. 1973. Psychiatric aspects of aphasia. 555-566.

Benson, D.F. 1979. *Aphasia, Alexia and Agraphia*. New York: Churchill Livingstone.

Benson, D.F. 1980. Psychiatric problems in aphasia. In: Sarno, M.T. and Höök, O. (Eds.,) *Aphasia: Assessment and Treatment*. Stockholm: Almqvist & Wiksell.

Benson, D.F. and Geschwind, N. 1983. The aphasias and related disturbances. In: Baker, A.B. and Baker, L.H. (Eds), *Clinical Neurology* Vol. 1. Philadelphia: Harper and Row.

Benton, A.L. 1968. Differential behavioral effects in frontal lobe disease. *Neuropsychologia* 6, 53-60.

Bertalanffy, L.V. 1968. *General System Theory*. New York: George Braziller.

Biorn-Hansen, V. 1957. Social and emotional aspects of aphasia. *Journal of Speech and Hearing Disorders* 22, 53-59.

Blackman, N. 1950. Group psychotherapy with aphasics. *The Journal of Nervous and Mental*

Disease 3, 154-163.

Bleuler, E.P. (1951) *Textbook of Psychiatry*. New York: Dover.

Borenstein, P., Linell, S. and Währborg, P. 1987. An innovative therapeutic program for aphasia patients and their relatives. *Scandinavian Journal of Rehabilitation Medicine* 19, 51-56.

Borenstein, P., Währborg, P., Linell, S., Hedberg, E., Asking, M. and Ahlsen, E. 1987. Education in Folk High School for younger aphasic people. *Aphasiology* 1, 263-266.

Bradley, J.V. 1968. *Distribution-Free Statistical Tests*. London: Prentice Hall.

Broca, P. 1861. Remarques sur le siége de la faculté du langage articulé, suives d'une observation d'aphemie. *Bull. Soc. Anat.* 36, 330-357.

Brooks, N., Campsie, L., Symington, C., Beattie, A. and McKinlay, W. 1986. The five year outcome of severe blunt head injury: a relative's view. *Journal of Neurology, Neurosurgery and Psychiatry* 49, 764-770.

Brown, J.W. 1988. *The Life of the Mind*. Hillsdale: LEA.

Brumfitt, S. and Clarke, P. 1989. An application of psychotherapeutic techniques to the management of aphasia. In: Code, C. & Müller, D.J., (Eds.,) *Aphasia Therapy* (2nd Edition). London: Whurr.

Cameron, H. 1959. Rationalizing aphasic personality. *American Association of Industrial Nurses Journal* 7 (July), 14.

Cannon, W.B. 1927. The James-Lange theory of emotion: a critical examination and an alternative theory. *American Journal of Psychology* 39, 106-124.

Caplan, D. (1987) *Neurolinguistics and Linguistic Aphasiology*. Cambridge: Cambridge University Press.

Carroll, B.J., Fielding, J.M. and Blahski, T.G. (1973) Depression rating scales: A critical review. *Archives of General Psychiatry* 28, 361-365.

Carroll, B.J., Curtis, G.C. and Mendels, J. 1976 a,b. Neuroendocrine regulation in depression. I. Limbic system-adrenocortical dysfunction. II. Discrimination of depressed from nondepressed patients. *Archives of General Psychiatry* 33, 1039 and 1051.

Carroll, B.J., Feinberg, M., Greden, J.F., Tarika, J., Albala, A.A., Haskett, R.F., James, N.M., Kronfol, Z., Lohr, N., Steiner, M, de Vigne, J.P. and Young, E. 1981. A specific laboratory test for the diagnosis of melancholia. *Archives of General Psychiatry* 38, 15-22.

Code, C. 1986. Catastrophic reactions and anosognosia in anterior-posterior and left-right models of the cerebral control of emotion. *Psychological Research* 48, 53-55.

Code, C. 1987. *Language, Aphasia and the Right Hemisphere*. Chichester: Wiley.

Code, C. (Ed.,) 1989. *The Characteristics of Aphasia*. Hove & London: Lawrence Erlbaum Associates.

Code, C. and Müller, D.J. (In Press) *The Code-Müller Protocols*. Kibworth: Far Communications.

Cooley, C.H. 1902. *Human Nature and the Social Order*. New York: Charles Scribner & Sons.

Cronholm, B. and Ottosson, J.O. 1960. Experimental studies of the therapeutic action of electroconvulsive therapy in endogenous depression. The role of the electric stimulation and the seizure studied by variation of stimulus intensity and modification by lidokain of seizure discharge. *Acta Psychiatrica Scandinavica* 35, Suppl. 145, 69.

Cullberg, J. (1975) *Kris Och Utveckling*. Stockholm: Natur & Kultur.

D'Afflitti, J.G. and Weitz, G.W. 1974. Rehabilitating the stroke patient: patient-family groups. *International Journal of Group Psychotherapy* 25, 323-332.

Dahlin, O. 1745. Berättelse om en dumbe som kan sjunga. In: *Kongliga Vetenskapsakademiens*. Handlingar, Stockholm.

Damasio, A. 1979. The frontal lobes. In: Heilman, K.M. and Valenstein, E. (Eds.,) *Clinical Neuropsychology*. Oxford: Oxford University Press.

Dana, C.S. 1921. The autonomic seat of the emotions: a discussion of the James-Lange theory. *Archives of Neurology and Psychiatry* 6, 634.

Davidson, R.J. 1983. Affect, cognition and hemispheric specialization. In: Izard, C.E., Kagan, J. and Zajonc, R. (Eds.,) *Emotion, Cognition and Behaviour*. Cambridge: Cambridge University Press.

Davis, K. 1947. Final note on a case of extreme isolation. *American Journal of Sociology* 52, 432-437.

Derman, S. and Manaster, A. 1967. Family counselling with relatives of aphasic patients at Schwab Rehabilitation Hospital. *Astra* 9, 175-177.

Diagnostic and Statistical Manual of Mental Disorders, 3rd Edition. (1980) Washington DC: American Psychiatric Association.

Emerson, R. 1980. Changes in depression and self-esteem of spouses of stroke patients with aphasia as a result of group-counselling. *Dissertation Abstracts International* Vol. 40, 4895.

Espmark, S. 1973 Stroke before 50. *Scandinavian Journal of Rehabilitation Medicine*, Suppl. 2.

Eysenck, H.J. and Eysenck, S.B.G. (1964) *Manual of the Eysenck Personality Inventory*. London: University of London Press.

Fiebel, J.H., Berk, S. and Joynt, R.J. 1979. The unmet needs of stroke survivors. *Neurology* 29, 592-594.

Finkelstein, S., Benowitz, L.J., Baldessarini, R.G., Arana, G.W. Levine, D., Woo, E., Bear, D., Moya, K. and Stoll, A.L. 1982. Mood, vegetative disorders and dexamethasone suppression test after stroke. *Annals of Neurology* 12, 463-468.

Fisher, S. 1961. Psychiatric considerations of cerebral vascular disease. *American Journal of Cardiology* 7, 379-383.

Flowers, C.R., Beukelman, D.R., Bottorf, L.E. and Kelley, R.A. 1979. Family members' predictions of aphasic test performance. *Aphasia, Apraxia, Agnosia* 1, 18-26.

Folstein, M.F., Folstein, S.F. and McHugh, P.R. 1975. Mini-Mental State: A practical method for grading the cognitive state of patients for the clinician. *Journal of Psychiatric Research* 12, 189-198

Folstein, M.F., Maiberger, R. and McHugh P.R. 1977. Mood disorder as a specific complication of stroke. *Journal of Neurology, Neurosurgery and Psychiatry* 40, 1018-1020.

References

Frank, J.D. 1972. Common features of psychotherapy. *Australian and New Zealand J of Psychiatry* 6, 34-43.

Friedman, M.H. 1961. On the nature of repression in aphasia. *Archives of General Psychiatry* 5, 252-256.

Gainotti, G. 1972. Emotional behavior and hemispheric side of lesion. *Cortex* 8, 41-45.

Gloning, I., Gloning, K., Haub, G. and Quatember, R. 1969. Comparison of verbal behavior in righthanded and non-righthanded patients with anatomically verified lesion of one hemisphere. *Cortex* 5, 43-53.

Goldstein, K. 1935. The modification of behavior consequent to cerebral lesions. *Psychiatry Quarterly* 10, 586-610.

Goldstein, K. 1939. *The Organism: A Holistic Approach to Biology Derived from Pathological Data in Man.* New York: American Books.

Goldstein, K. 1942. *After Effects of Brain Injuries in War.* New York: Grune & Stratton.

Goldstein, K. 1948. *Language and Language Disturbance.* New York: Grune & Stratton.

Goodglass, H. and Kaplan, E. 1972. *The Assessment of Aphasia and Related Disorders.* Philadelphia: Lea & Febiger.

Haese, J.B. 1970. Attitudes of stroke patients toward rehabilitation and recovery. *American Journal of Occupational Therapy* 24, 4-11.

Haley, J. 1962. Family experiments: A new type of experimentations. *Family Process* 1, 265-398.

Hamilton, M.A. 1960. A Rating Scale for Depression. *Journal of Neurology, Neurosurgery and Psychiatry* 23, 56-62.

Hansson, K. (1989) Familjediagnostik. *Akademisk avhandling, Institutionen för barn- och ungdomspsykiatri.* Lunds Universitet, Lund.

Hécaen, H. 1967. Brain mechanisms suggested by studies of parietal lobes. In: Millikan, C.H. and Darley, F.L. (Eds.,) *Brain Mechanisms Underlying Speech and Language.* New York: Grune & Stratton.

Hedberg-Borenstein, E., Währborg, P., Gustavsson, I., Jensson, A. and Borenstein, P. 1988. A comparison between aphasia testing outcome and the ability of aphasics and their spouses to judge language ability. In: Währborg, P. (Ed.,) *After Stroke - Behavioral changes and therapeutic intervention in aphasics and their relatives following stroke.* Thesis, Gothenburg: University of Gothenburg.

Helmick, J.W., Watamori, T.S. and Palmer, J.M. 1976. Spouses understanding of the communication disabilities of aphasic patients. *Journal of Speech and Hearing Disorders* 41, 238-272.

Helmick, J.W., Watamori, T.S. and Palmer, J.M. 1977. Reply to Holland's comment on "Spouses understanding of the communication disabilities of aphasic patients". *Journal of Speech and Hearing Disorders* 42, 308-310.

Herrmann, M. and Wallesch, C-W. 1990. Expectations of psychosocial adjustment in aphasia: a MAUT study with the Code-Müller Scale of Psychosocial Adjustment. *Aphasiology* 4, 527-538.

Holland, A. (1977) Comment on spouses understanding of the communication disabilities of aphasic patients. *Journal of Speech and Hearing Disorders* 42, 307-308.

Höök, O. 1979. Aphasia and related communication disorders after brain injury. *Paper presented at the Second Annual Conference: Head Trauma Rehabilitation, Coma to Community.* San Jose, California, USA.

James, W. (1884) What is an emotion? *Mind* 9, 188-196.

Jenkins, J., Jiménez-Pabón, E., Shaw, R.E. and Sefer, J.W. (1975) *Schuell's Aphasia in Adults.* New York: Harper & Row.

Jung, R. 1974. Neuropsychologie und Neurophysiologie des konturend Formsehens in Zeichnung und Malerei. In: Wieck, H.H. *Psychopathologie musischer Gestaltungen.* Stuttgart: F.K. Schattauer Verlag.

Kinsella, G.J. and Duffy, F. 1978. The spouse of the aphasic patient. In: Lebrun, Y. and Hoops, R. (Eds.,) *The Management of Aphasia.* Amsterdam: Swets and Zeitlinger.

Kinsella, G.J. and Duffy, F. 1979. Psychosocial adjustment in the spouses of aphasic patients. *Scandinavian Journal of Rehabilitation Medicine* 11, 129-132.

Klüver, H. and Bucy, P.C. 1939. Preliminary analysis of functions of the temporal lobes in monkeys. *Archives of Neurology and Psychiatry* 42, 979-1000.

Knesevich, J.W., Biggs, J.T., Clayton, P.J. and Ziegler, V.E. 1977. Validity of the Hamilton Rating Scale for Depression. *British Journal of Psychiatry* 131, 49-55.

Kraepelin, E. 1921. *Manic Depressive Insanity and Paranoia.* Edinburgh: E&S Livingstone.

Kubler-Ross, E. 1969. *On Death and Dying.* New York: MacMillan.

Kurtzke, J.F. 1982. The current neurologic burden of illness and injury in the United States. *Neurology* 11, 686.

Lashley, K. 1929. *Brain Mechanisms and Intelligence.* Chicago: University of Chicago Press.

Laurence, S. and Stein, D.G. 1978. Recovery after brain damage and the concept of localization of function. In: Finger, S. (Ed.,) *Recovery from Brain Damage.* New York: Plenum Press.

Lichtheim, L. 1885. Über aphasie. *Deutches Archiv. für Klin. Med.* 36, 204-268.

Linell, S and Steg, G. 1980. Family treatment in aphasia - experience from a patient association. In: Taylor-Sarno, M. and Höök, O. (Eds.,) *Aphasia, Assessment and Treatment.* Stockholm: Almqvist & Wiksell International.

Lincoln, N.B., Jones, A.C. and Mulley, G.P. 1985. Psychological effects of speech therapy. *Journal of Psychosomatic Research* 29, 467-474.

Lipowski, Z.J. 1974. Physical illness, the patient and his environment: psychosocial foundations of medicine. In: Arieti, S. (Ed.,) *American Handbook of Psychiatry* Vol. 4. New York: Basic Books.

Lipsey, J.R., Robinson, R.G., Pearlson, G.D., Rao, K. and Price, T.R. 1984. Nortriptyline treatment of post-stroke depression: A double-blind study. *The Lancet* 11 (February), 297-300.

Lipsey, J.R., Robinson, R.G., Pearlson, G.D., Rao, K. and Price, T.R. 1985. Dexamethasone suppression test and mood following stroke. *American Journal of Psychiatry* 142, 318-323.

Lipsey, J.R., Spencer, W.C., Rabins, P.V. and Robinson, R.G. 1986. Phenomenological

References

comparison of post-stroke depression and functional depression. *American Journal of Psychiatry* 143, 527-529.

Louis, S. and McDowell, F. 1967. Epileptic seizures in non-embolic cerebral infarction. *Archives of Neurology* 17, 414.

Lundholm, J., Jepsen, B.N. and Thornval, G. 1975. The late neurological, psychological and social aspects of severe traumatic coma. *Scandinavian Journal of Rehabilitation Medicine* 7, 97-100.

Lundsbye, M, Sandell, G., Währborg, P., Ferm, R. and Petitt, B. 1982. *Familjeterapins Grunder.* Stockholm: Natur & Kultur.

Luria, A.R. 1973. *The Working Brain.* Harmondsworth: Penguin.

MacDonald, M.R., Nielson, W.R. and Cameron, M.G.P. 1987. Depression and activity patterns of spinal cord injured persons living in the community. *Archives of Physical Medicine Rehabilitation* 68, 393-347.

Malone, R.L. 1969. Expressed attitudes of families of aphasics. *Journal of Speech and Hearing Disorders* 34, 146-151.

Malone, R.L., Ptacek, P.H. and Malone, M.S. 1970. Attitudes expressed by families of aphasics. *British Journal of Disorders of Communication* 5, 174-179.

Mapelli, G., Pavoni, M. and Ramelli, E. 1980. Emotional and psychotic reactions induced by aphasia. *Psychiatria Clinica* 13, 108-118.

Maas, J.W. 1975. Biogenic amines and depression. Biochemical and pharmacological separation of two types of depression. *Archives of General Psychiatry* 32, 1357-1361.

Mead, G.H. 1934. *Mind, Self and Society.* London: The University of Chicago Press.

Meyer, A. 1904. The anatomical facts and clinical varieties of traumatic insanity. *American Journal of Insanity* 60, 373.

Milner, B. 1967. Comments on Rossi and Rosadini. In: Millikan, C.H. and Darley, F.L. (Eds.,) *Brain Mechanisms Underlying Speech and Language.* New York: Grune & Stratton.

Monakow, C.V. 1914. *Die Lokalisation im Grosshirnrinde unter der Abban der Funktion durch Korticale Herde.* Wiesbaden: J.F. Bergman.

Montgomery, S., Asberg, M., Jörnestedt, L, Thorén, P., Träskman, L., McAuley, R., Montgomery, D. and Shaw, P. 1978. Reliability of the CPRS between the disciplines of psychiatry, general practice, nursing and psychology in depressed patients. *Acta Psychiatrica Scandinavica.* Suppl. 271.

Mountcastle, V.B. 1975. The view from within: pathways to the study of perception. *John Hopkins Medical Journal* 136, 109-115.

Mulhall, D.J. 1977. The representation of personal relationships: an automated system. *International Journal of Man-Machine Studies* 9, 315-335.

Mulhall, D.J. 1978. Dysphasic stroke patients and the influence of their relatives. *British Journal of Disorders of Communication* 13, 127-134.

Mulhall, D.J. 1979. *A systems approach to personal interaction in health care.* Paper presented at the Twenty-Fourth North American Annual Meeting of the Society for General Systems Research. Houston, Texas.

Müller, D.J., Code, C. and Mugford, J. 1983. Predicting psychosocial adjustment to aphasia.

British Journal of Disorders of Communication 18, 23-29.

Müller, D.J. and Code, C. 1989. Interpersonal perceptions of psychosocial adjustment to aphasia. In: Code, C. and Müller, D.J. (Eds.,) *Aphasia Therapy* (2nd Edition). London: Whurr.

Murdoch, B. 1989. *Acquired Speech & Language Disorders*. London: Chapman & Hall

Najenson, T., Mendelson; L., Schechter, I, David, C., Minz, N. and Groswasser, Z. 1974. Rehabilitation after severe head injury. *Scandinavian Journal of Rehabilitation Medicine* 6, 5-14.

Oster, C. 1976. Sensory deprivation in geriatric patients. *Journal of the American Geriatrics Society*. 24, 461-463.

Overs, R.P. and Healy, J. 1971. Educating stroke patient families. *Milwaukee Media for Rehabilitation Research Reports* 12 (July).

Papez, J.W. 1937. A proposed mechanism of emotion. *Archives of Neurology and Psychiatry* 38, 725-743.

Parikh, R.M., Lipsey, J.R., Robinson, R.G. and Price, T.R. 1987. Two year longitudinal study of post-stroke mood disorders: dynamic changes in correlates of depression at one and two years. *Stroke* 18, 579-584

Popper, K.R. 1977. In: Popper, K.R. and Eccles, J.C. *The Self and Its Brain.* Berlin: Springer International.

Porch, B.E. 1967a. *Porch Index of Communicative Ability. Vol.I: Theory and Development.* Palo Alto: Consulting Psychologists.

Porch, B.E. 1967b. *Porch Index of Communicative Ability. Vol.II: Administration, Scoring and Interpretation.* Palo Alto: Consulting Psychologists.

Powell, G. E. 1981. *Brain Function Therapy.* Aldershot: Gower.

Reding, M.J., Orto, L. A., Willenski, P., Fortuna, I., Day, N., Steiner, S.F., Gehr, L. and McDowell, F. 1985. The dexamethasone suppression test is an indicator of depression in stroke but does not predict rehabilitation outcome. *Archives of Neurology* 42, 209-212.

Reding, M.J., Orto, L.A., Winter, S.W., Fortuna, I.M., Di Ponte, P. and McDowell, F.H. 1986. Antidepressant therapy After stroke: a double blind trial. *Archives of Neurology* 43, 763-765.

Reinvang, I. and Engvik, H. 1980. *Norsk grunntest for afasi.* (Swedish translation by P Borenstein). Oslo: Universitetsforlaget.

Reitan, R.M. and Davison, L.A. (1974) *Clinical Neuropsychology: Current status and Applications.* New York: John Wiley.

Ricco-Schwartz, S. 1982. Fostering an empathic approach: an in-service curriculum for nonmedical professionals, paraprofessionals and families of aphasic clients. *Gerontology and Geriatrics Education* 2, 199-206.

Rice, B., Paull, A. and Müller, D.J. 1987. An evaluation of a social support group for spouses of aphasic partners. *Aphasiology* 1, 247-256.

Roach, A., Frazier, L.P and Bowden, S.R. 1981. Marital satisfaction scale: development of a measure for intervention research. *Journal of Marriage and Family* 43, 537-546.

References

Robinson, R.G. and Benson, D.F. 1981. Depression in aphasic patients: frequency severity and clinical-pathological correlations. *Brain and Language* 14, 282-291.

Robinson, R.G., Kubos, K.L., Starr, L.B., Rao, K. and Price, T.R. 1984. Mood disorders in stroke patients: importance of location of lesion. *Brain* 107, 81-93.

Robinson, R.G. and Price, T.R. 1982. Post-stroke depressive disorders: a follow-up study of 103 patients. *Stroke* 13, 635-640.

Robinson, R.G., Starr, L.B. and Price, T.R. 1984. A two year longitudinal study of mood disorders following stroke: prevalence and duration at six months follow up. *British Journal of Psychiatry* 144, 256-264.

Robinson, R.G. and Szetala, B. 1981. Mood change following left hemispheric brain injury. *Annals of Neurology* 3, 447-453.

Rollin, W. 1988. Family therapy and the aphasic adult. In: Eisenson, J. (Ed.,) *Adult Aphasia.* Englewood Cliffs, N.J.: Prentice-Hall.

Ross, E. D. & Rush, J.A. 1981. Diagnosis and neuroanatomical correlates of depression in brain-damaged patients. *Archives of General Psychiatry* 38, 1344-1354.

Rossi, G.F., & Rosadini, G. 1967. Experimental analysis of cerebral dominance in man. In: C.H. Millikan and F.L. Darley (eds.), *Brain Mechanisms Underlying Speech and Language.* New York: Grune & Stratton.

Rubenowitz, S. 1977. *Hamilton's bedömningsschema för depressiva tillständ.* Goteborg: Lillhagens Sjukhus.

Sackeim, H.A., Greenberg, M.S., Weiman, A.L., Gur, R.C., Hungerbuhler, J.P. and Geschwind, N. 1982. Hemispheric asymmetry in the expression of positive and negative emotions: neurological evidence. *Archives of Neurology* 39, 210-218.

Satir, V. (1976) *Making Contact.* Millbrae: Celestial Arts.

Schatzman, M. 1974. *Soul Murder, Persecution in the Family.* New York: The New American Library.

Schildkraut, J.J. 1965. The catecholamine hypothesis of affective disorders: a review of supporting evidence. *American Journal of Psychiatry* 122, 509-522.

Schwartz, G.E., Davidson, R.J. and Maer, F. 1975. Right hemisphere lateralization for emotion in the human brain: interactions with cognition. *Science* 190, 286.

Sinyor, D., Jacques, P., Kaloupek, D.B., Becker, R., Goldenberg, M. and Coopersmith, H.M. 1986. Post-stroke depression and lesion location: an attempted replication. *Brain* 109, 537-546.

Soltero, I., Kiang Liu, Cooper, R., Stamlel, J. and Garside, D. 1978. Trends in mortality from cerebrovascular diseases in the United States 1960-1975. *Stroke* 9, 549-649.

Starkstein, S.E. and Robinson, R.G. 1988. Aphasia and depression, *Aphasiology* 2, 1-20

Svennerholm, L. 1989. Personal Communication.

Tanner, D.C. and Gerstenberger, D.L. 1988. The grief response in neuropathologies of speech and language. *Aphasiology* 2, 79-84.

Taylor, M. 1965. A measurement of functional communication in aphasia. *Archives of Physical Medicine Rehabilitation* 46, 101-107.

Taylor, M. 1969. *Understanding Aphasia.* American Heart Association.

Taylor-Sarno, M. (Ed.,) 1981. *Acquired Aphasia.* New York: Academic Press.

Terzian, H. and Ceccotto, C. 1959. Su di un nuovo metodo per la determinazione e lo studio della dominanza emisferica. *Psichiatrica Neuropathologica* 57, 889-923.

Thompson, G.N. 1948. Fear reaction induced by aphasia. *Bulletin of the Los Angeles Neurological Society* 13. 233-270.

Thomsen, I.V. 1984. Late outcome of very severe blunt head trauma: a 10-15 year second follow up. *Journal of Neurology, Neurosurgery and Psychiatry* 47, 260-268.

Tucker, D.M. 1981. Lateral brain function, emotion, and conceptualization. *Psychological Bulletin* 89, 19-46.

Turnblom, M. and Myers, J.S. 1952. A group discussion program with the families of aphasic patients. *Journal of Speech and Hearing Disorders* 17, 393-396.

Ullman, M. 1962. *Behavioural Changes in Patients Following Strokes.* Springfield, Ill: Charles C. Thomas.

Währborg, P. and Borenstein, P. 1987. *Depression after stroke, some nosological considerations.* Proceedings, First European Conference on Aphasiology. Vienna: Austrian Workers' Compensation Board.

Walrond-Skinner, S. 1976. *Family Therapy.* London: Routledge & Kegan Paul.

Währborg, P. 1989. Aphasia and family therapy. *Aphasiology* 3, 479-482.

Währborg, P. 1990. The aphasic person and his/her family: what about the future. *Aphasiology* 4, 371-378.

Währborg, P. and Borenstein, P. 1988a. Behavioral changes after stroke. In: Währborg, P. *After Stroke - Behavioral changes and therapeutic intervention in aphasics and their relatives following stroke.* Thesis, Gothenburg: University of Gothenburg.

Währborg, P. and Borenstein, P. 1988b. Progressive psychological deterioration in aphasic and non-aphasic stroke patients. In: Währborg, P. *After Stroke - Behavioral changes and therapeutic intervention in aphasics and their relatives following stroke.* Thesis, Gothenburg: University of Gothenburg.

Währborg, P. and Borenstein, P. 1989. Family therapy in families with an aphasic member. *Aphasiology* 3, 93-97.

Watzlawick, P., Beavin, J.H. and Jackson, D.D. 1967. *Pragmatics of Human Communication.* New York: W.W. Norton & Co.

Wepman, J. 1951. *Recovery from Aphasia.* New York: Ronald.

Wernicke, C. 1874. *Der aphasiche symtomenkomplex.* Breslau: Cohn und Weigert.

World Health Organization 1980. *International Classification of Impairments, Disabilities and Handicaps.* Geneva: World Health Organization.

Williams, S.E. and Freer, C.A. 1986. Aphasia: its effect on marital relationships. *Archives of Physical Medicine Rehabilitation* 67, 250-252.

Woolsey, T.A. 1978. Lesion experiments: some anatomical considerations. In: Finger, S. (Ed.,) *Recovery from Brain Damage.* New York: Plenum Press.

Zubek, J.P. 1974. Sensory isolation: fifteen years of research at the University of Manitoba. *Studia Psychologica* 16, 265-274.

Zung, W.K. 1965. A self-rating depression scale. *Archives of General Psychiatry* 12-70.

Anosognosia 16, 17
Assessment 1-5, 13, 49, 55, 58-60, 64,
     66, 68, 69, 103
  biochemical data 55
Barthel activities of daily living 98
Behavioural changes in aphasia 5, 8-
     12, 14, 47, 73, 100

CMP see *Code-Müller Protocols*
Code-Müller Protocols (CMP) 33, 64-
     65
Comprehensive Psychopathological
     Rating Scale (CPRS) 61, 62,
     93, 96, 97
Cooperation 53
CPRS see *Comprehensive
     Psychopathological Rating
     Scale*

Depression
  major post-stroke depression
          20, 23, 24, 57
  reactive post-stroke
          depression 20, 23
Depression and the hemispheres 16,
     18
Depression Scales 60-62
  Beck Depression Inventory
          60-62
  Hamilton Depression Scale 5,
          10, 60-62
  Zung 60-62
Disability 10, 48, 52, 70-72

Euphoria 8, 54

Family assessment 68, 69
Family diagnosis 49, 67, 68
Family dynamics 67, 68
Family therapy 39, 69, 74, 76, 80-86

Group therapy 86-88

Interaction 6, 11, 39, 41, 42, 44,
     45, 65-67
Knowledge of aphasia, patient and
     family 33, 34, 76
Long-term evolution of emotional
     state 5, 99

Management 1-5, 40, 70, 103
Marital Satisfaction Scale 34, 69

Observations 3, 6, 9, 10, 15, 17,
     33, 47, 50, 52, 54, 55, 114
Patient associations in
     management 78

Pharmological treatment 98
Personal Relations Index (PRI) 65,
     66, 79
PRI see *Personal Relations Scale*
Programme for young aphasic
     adults 93
Projection 12, 43, 44, 54, 91
Psychiatric disorders 11, 12, 25,
     33, 39, 48, 57
  agitation 12, 20, 39, 61
  anxiety reactions 12, 39
  guilt feelings 32, 39, 54, 61
Psychotherapy 12, 39, 78-80,
     86-90

Questionnaires in assessment 7,
     13, 14, 57, 58, 63, 64, 85

Rating Scales 59, 61, see also
     Depression scales
Recovery from brain damage 72
  denervation 73
  diaschisis 47, 73
  ineffective synapses 73

Residential programmes in
        management 74
Right hemisphere, role in cognition
        and behaviour 13, 16-18, 21,
        53
Scientific methods 7
Self, development of 41, 42
    interpersonal interaction 45
    projection 44
    the physical system 45, 46
    the representational system
            41
Socialization 42, 45, 67, 114
Support programmes 78, 79-80

Tests 2, 7, 35, 57, 58, 79
    reliability 59, 61-63
    standardization 58, 63
    validity 58, 59, 62, 63
The examination 50, 55
    the interview 50, 51, 63, 82,
            85
    systematic observations 52
The grief reaction 90-92
Therapy 24, 30-32, 39, 69, 74-76, 78,
        80-83, 85, 86, 89, 90, 98
Treatment 25, 48, 53, 55, 56, 70, 73,
        74, 87-89, 97, 98
Unilateral neglect 17

VAS see *Visual Analogue Scale*
Visual Analogue Scale (VAS) 12, 20,
        36, 37, 39, 59, 60, 61, 62
World Health Organization International
        Classification of Disability 70,
        71
    disability 71
    handicap 71
    impairment 70